# OVERVIEW M[...]

## :: OTHER TITLES IN THIS SERIES

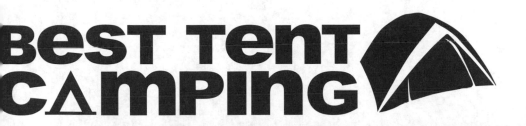

# BEST TENT CAMPING
# NEW MEXICO

## YOUR CAR-CAMPING GUIDE TO SCENIC BEAUTY, THE SOUNDS OF NATURE, AND AN ESCAPE FROM CIVILIZATION

2nd Edition

# MONTE R. PARR

MENASHA RIDGE PRESS
*Your Guide to the Outdoors Since 1982*

**::** *This book is dedicated to my lovely wife, Susan Sherwood Parr. Thank you for all the encouragement and support, and especially our adventures in the wilderness together.*

**Best Tent Camping: New Mexico, 2nd Edition**

Copyright © 2014 by Monte R. Parr
All rights reserved
Printed in the United States of America
Published by Menasha Ridge Press
Distributed by Publishers Group West
Second edition, first printing

Library of Congress Cataloging-in-Publication Data

Parr, Monte Russ.
  Best tent camping, New Mexico : your car-camping guide to scenic beauty, the sounds of nature, and an escape from civilization / Monte Parr.
    pages cm
  ISBN 978-0-89732-502-8 (paperback) — ISBN 0-89732-502-8
  1.  Camp sites, facilities, etc.—New Mexico—Directories. 2.  Camping—New Mexico—Guidebooks. 3.  New Mexico—Guidebooks.  I. Title.
  GV191.42.N6P37 2014
  796.5409789—dc23
                    2014013745

Cover design by Scott McGrew
Cover photo © CWLawrence
Cartography by Steve Jones and Monte R. Parr
Indexing by Rich Carlson

Menasha Ridge Press
P.O. Box 43673
Birmingham, Alabama 35243
menasharidge.com

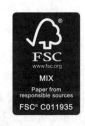

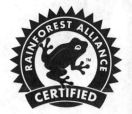

# CONTENTS

## :: SOUTHEASTERN NEW MEXICO   95

## :: SOUTHWESTERN NEW MEXICO   133

## :: APPENDIXES   164

# BEST CAMPGROUNDS

•  •  •  •  •  •  •  •  •  •  •  •  •  •  •  •  •  •  •  •  •  •  •  •

## :: BEST FOR WHEELCHAIRS

# ACKNOWLEDGMENTS

● ● ● ● ● ● ● ● ● ● ● ● ● ● ● ● ● ● ● ● ● ● ● ●

**I wish to** express my deepest heartfelt gratitude to the following people for their love, kindness, support, encouragement, and friendship: my wife, Susan Sherwood Parr; my dear stepson, Chris Livingston; my brother, Robert, and Debra Parr; the entire Sherwood family; and Pastor Eric and Debbie Larson. Thanks to Peter Benson and Steve Reimann at KNKT 707.1 Connection Radio for their interest in my projects and for airtime.

Many thanks to Molly Merkle and all the kind folks at Menasha Ridge Press for their input, professional skills, and encouragement. They have no idea what an adventure they have given me. I am grateful and humbled to be chosen as the author for this book.

My gratitude also goes to the members of the following government agencies: Mescalero Apache Nation, National Park Service, New Mexico County Sheriff's Departments, New Mexico Department of Game and Fish, New Mexico State Parks, New Mexico State Police, United States Army Corps of Engineers, United States Bureau of Land Management, United States Fish and Wildlife Service, and United States Forest Service. These folks were friendly, helpful, and informative. Without their assistance, this project could not have been completed.

I would also like to thank the following businesses for their help and inspiration with this project: Amanda's General Store, Der Markt Food Store, Manzano Tiendita, Ray's General Store, Sportsmen's Warehouse, The Sherwood Company, and Word Productions.

# PREFACE

● ● ● ● ● ● ● ● ● ● ● ● ● ● ● ● ● ● ● ● ● ● ●

**I have loved** the outdoors since I was knee-high to a short toad. I was raised by my grandparents, who taught me to slow down, be observant, and appreciate the gifts Mother Nature has generously given all of us. I was like most kids; I started camping in the backyard, with a sheet draped over the clothesline, sleeping on an old Army cot and sleeping bag. In high school, I spent many hours hiking the hundreds of acres of hardwood forests behind our home in Iowa with a knapsack, a sleeping bag, and an old Army pup tent.

My early adult life was spent backpacking and car camping the wonderful state parks throughout Nebraska. I moved to Colorado for two years and continued backpacking and car camping the high country. I moved to New Mexico in August of 1988, and the next weekend I launched my first trip into the Jemez Wilderness. It was there that I discovered the Land of Enchantment was where I was destined to be.

I am convinced that tent camping is the purest and most rewarding method of experiencing nature. During high winds, drenching downpours, and lightning storms, tent camping is a challenge, but I prefer tent camping to RV camping. On a brightly moonlit night, I love the shadows of the tree branches dancing on the roof of the tent. I love to watch the campfire flames and glowing embers. I love going to sleep with the sounds of a night bird calling, the hooting of an owl from deep in the forest, and the distant howl of the coyote.

I love the sound of the mountain breeze as it catches the upper branches of a giant ponderosa—wind gusting through ponderosa pine trees sounds like the ocean surf rushing to the shore. You can hear the creaking of the branches and watch the camber of the tree as it bends in the wind.

It is a healthy choice to escape the electronic paraphernalia that inundates our society and all the stresses that come with technology. I leave the gadgets at home. It seems the simpler you camp, the more you enjoy the experience. When I started camping, I used an old saucepan and a roll of foil and cooked over the fire like a cowboy. When I bought a cookstove and lantern, I thought I was in hog heaven!

When I began this project, I had absolutely no clue what a delightful undertaking it would be. This opportunity has allowed me to visit every county in New Mexico, every national forest, and all of the major historical areas the 47th state offers. I traveled in excess of 9,000 miles and visited more than 160 campgrounds. The majority of them deserve a profile in this book; eliminating many deserving campgrounds was difficult but inevitable.

It is my sincere wish that this book will enhance your camping experiences in New Mexico, and that you experience all the joys and blessings in your travels that I have.

Respectfully,
*Monte R. Parr*

# INTRODUCTION

● ● ● ● ● ● ● ● ● ● ● ● ● ● ● ● ● ● ● ● ● ● ●

## How to Use This Guidebook

**We at Menasha Ridge Press** welcome you to *Best Tent Camping: New Mexico.* Whether you're new to this activity or you've been sleeping in your portable outdoor shelter over decades of outdoor adventures, please review the following information. It explains how we have worked with the author to organize this book and how you can make the best use of it.

Some passages in this introduction apply to all of the books in the *Best Tent Camping* guidebook series. Where this isn't the case, such as in the descriptions of weather, wildlife, and plants, the author has provided information specific to your area.

### :: THE RATINGS & RATING CATEGORIES

As with all of the books in the *Best Tent Camping* series, this guidebook's author personally experienced dozens of campgrounds and campsites to select the top 50 locations in this state. Within that universe of 50 sites, the author then ranked each one in the six categories described below. Each campground in this guidebook is superlative in its own way. For example, a site may be rated only one star in one category but perhaps five stars in another category. This rating system allows you to choose your destination based on the attributes that are most important to you.

★ ★ ★ ★ ★  The site is **ideal** in that category.
★ ★ ★ ★  The site is **exemplary** in that category.
★ ★ ★  The site is **very good** in that category.
★ ★  The site is **above average** in that category.
★  The site is **acceptable** in that category.

### *Beauty*

In the best campgrounds, the fluid shapes and elements of nature—flora, water, land, and sky—have melded to create locales that seem to have been made for tent camping. The best sites are so attractive that you may be tempted not to leave your outdoor home. A little site work is all right to make the scenic area camper-friendly, but too many reminders of civilization eliminated many a campground from inclusion in this book.

### *Privacy*

A little understory goes a long way in making you feel comfortable once you've picked your site for the night. There is a trend in planting natural borders between campsites if the borders don't exist already. With some trees or brush to define the sites, everyone has his or her personal space. Then you can go about the pleasures of tent camping without keeping up with the Joneses at the site next door—or them with you.

## Spaciousness

This attribute can be very important depending on how much of a gearhead you are and the size of your group. Campers with family-style tents and screen shelters need a large, flat spot on which to pitch a tent, with more room for the ice chest and to prepare foods, all the while not getting burned near the fire ring. We just want enough room to keep our bedroom, den, and kitchen separate.

## Quiet

When I go camping I want to hear the music of the lakes, rivers, and all the land between—the singing birds, rushing streams, and wind whooshing through the trees. In concert, these sounds camouflage the sounds you don't want to hear—autos coming and going, loud neighbors, and so on. Criteria for this rating include several touchstones: my experience at the site, the nearness of roads, the proximity of towns and cities, the probable number of RVs, the likelihood of noisy ATVs or boats, and whether a campground host is available or willing to enforce the quiet hours. Of course, one set of noisy neighbors can deflate a five-star rating into a one-star (or no-star), so the latter criterion—campground enforcement—was particularly important in the evaluations of this category.

## Security

How you determine a campground's security will depend on whom (or *what*) you view as the greater risk: other people or the wilderness. The more remote the campground, the less likely you are to run into opportunistic crime, but the more remote the campground, the harder it is to get help in case of an accident or dangerous wildlife confrontation. A remote campground with no civilization nearby is usually safe, but don't tempt potential thieves by leaving your valuables out for all to see. Campground hosts are wonderful to have around, and state parks with locked gates are ideal for security. Get to know your neighbors and develop a buddy system to watch each other's belongings when possible.

Ratings in this category take into consideration whether there was a campground host or resident park ranger, the proximity of other campers' sites, how much day traffic the campground received, how close the campground was to a town or city, and whether there was cell-phone reception or some type of pay phone or emergency call button.

## Cleanliness

Nothing will sabotage a scenic campground like trash. Most of the campgrounds in this guidebook are clean. More rustic campgrounds—our favorites—usually receive less maintenance. Busy weekends and holidays will show their effects; however, don't let a little litter spoil your good time. Help clean up, and think of it as doing your part for the environment.

A campground's appearance often depends on who was there right before you and how your visit coincides with the maintenance schedule. In general, higher marks went to those campgrounds with hosts who cleaned up regularly. The rare case of odor-free toilets also gleaned high marks. At campgrounds without a host, criteria included trash receptacles and evidence that sites were cleared and that signs and buildings were kept repaired. Markdowns for the campground were not given for a single visitor's garbage left at a site, but old trash in the shrubbery and along trails, indicating infrequent cleaning, did secure low ratings.

## :: THE CAMPGROUND PROFILE

Each profile contains a concise but informative narrative of the campground and individual sites. Not only is the property described, but also readers can get a general idea of the recreational opportunities available—what's in the area and perhaps suggestions for touristy activities. This descriptive text is enhanced with three helpful sidebars: Ratings, Key Information, and Getting There (accurate driving directions that lead you to the campground from the nearest major roadway, along with GPS coordinates).

## :: THE OVERVIEW MAP AND MAP KEY

Use the overview map on the inside front cover to pinpoint the location of each campground. The campground's number follows it throughout this guidebook: from the overview map, to the map key, to the table of contents, and to the profile's first page.

## :: CAMPGROUND-LAYOUT MAPS

Each profile contains a detailed map of campground sites, internal roads, facilities, and other key items. A map legend that details the symbols found on the campground-layout maps appears on the inside back cover.

## :: GPS CAMPGROUND-ENTRANCE COORDINATES

Readers can easily access all campgrounds in this book by using the directions given and the overview map, which shows at least one major road leading into the area. But for those who enjoy using GPS technology to navigate, the book includes coordinates for each campground's entrance in latitude and longitude, expressed in degrees and decimal minutes.

**GPS COORDINATES**   N36° 33.027'   W106° 20.693'

To convert GPS coordinates from degrees, minutes, and seconds to the above degrees–decimal minutes format, the seconds are divided by 60. For more on GPS technology, visit **usgs.gov.**

# About This Book

**Welcome to New Mexico, the Land of Enchantment!** Our beloved state is a diverse land of contrasts—of canyons, deserts, mesas, high mountains, rivers, lakes, and glorious sunsets. This is a magnificent state in which to experience the best in tent camping.

New Mexico is the fifth-largest state in the nation, with 121,655 square miles of land mass. Our population ranks 36th in the nation, with 2 million people. It ranks 45th in population density, with slightly fewer than 15 people per square mile.

The mountains of New Mexico aren't as high as neighboring Colorado's peaks, but our mountains are as breathtaking as any on the planet. Wheeler Peak, at 13,161 feet, is the highest of six summits above 13,000 feet. There are 32 peaks over 12,000 feet, and 37 mountains tower over 11,000 feet.

New Mexico has five national forests: Carson, Santa Fe, Cibola, Gila, and Lincoln. The Bureau of Land Management has divided New Mexico into seven field offices to manage public lands: Farmington, Rio Puerco, Socorro, Las Cruces, Taos, Roswell, and Carlsbad. New Mexico features 36 state parks with a diverse landscape of lakes, mountains, canyons, forests, deserts, and historical sites. More than 30 hot springs scattered throughout the state attract many naturalists (with and without bathing attire), and many of these hot springs are located near campgrounds. Without question, you will find dozens of campgrounds you will wish to revisit.

Often you will spot large elk herds grazing in high-country grasslands. Also look for mountain lions, bobcats, black bears, mule deer, buffalo, pronghorn antelope, wild mustangs, wild burros, coyotes, Mexican gray wolves, javelinas, and ringtail cats—just a few species of wildlife native to our state.

The bird population in New Mexico is enormous, with more species than most birdwatchers can identify. The Rio Grande River Valley south of Socorro, New Mexico, is on the migratory flyway, and several protected waterfowl habitats are nearby. We are blessed with a large population of hummingbirds, so you might want to bring a feeder—they are delightful little visitors to your camp and easy to photograph.

Canyon walls rise dramatically from valley floors, providing breeding habitat for bald and golden eagles, various species of hawks, and peregrine falcons. Mesa walls tell the geologic history of this state with exposed stratum of rock, lava, clay, and sandstone in colorful contrasts that cannot be described in words. Some mesa walls are painted green, with piñon, juniper, and cedar trees clinging to their steep sides.

Every spring the cacti bloom in vibrant colors under the bright Chihuahuan desert sun. Knee-high silver sage paints the desert floor with a silvery green landscape. Beautiful yucca plant stalks bloom with shoots filled with white flowers. Greasewood, creosote, and mesquite shrubs are common throughout the desert. In the mountains, wildflowers of every color explode in springtime and stay until frost appears in the fall. Arroyos fill with rainwater and pour over the parched land as the monsoon season arrives in July. The thirsty deserts and Sangre de Cristo Mountains drink in the moisture and become lush and green. In autumn, aspen, oak, cottonwood, and willow trees explode in bright oranges, yellows, and reds, painting the mountains, valleys, and river basins.Winter snows begin in November. Skiers arrive at the slopes and resorts dotting the state. Snowbirds escaping the harsh winters of the northern states also arrive in November across the southern half of New Mexico. They feed the economies of dozens of towns through the month of April.

South of Truth or Consequences, New Mexico, the Mesilla (pronounced meh–SEE–yuh) Valley is a glorious contrast of green adjacent to the brown Turtle and Caballo Mountains to the east and brown desert to the west. The Mesilla Valley follows the Rio Grande River from north of Hatch, New Mexico, all the way south to El Paso, Texas. Since the valley is quite fertile, agriculture is the primary activity in this area. Just about every vegetable you can imagine is grown here, notably the Vidalia and Mayan sweet onions. The world's largest pecan orchard is located in the valley, and the area is famous for its pistachio nuts. Fruit orchards produce apples, peaches, plums, and other fruit. And the world-famous New Mexico green and red chiles are grown here and shipped worldwide.

Many geologic wonders abound in New Mexico: Tent Rocks, La Ventana Arch, Echo Amphitheatre, Valley of Fires, El Malpais, Chimney Rock, Carlsbad Caverns, and the Taos Gorge are just a few. Six state and 13 national monuments provide diverse educational, historical, and cultural experiences. Bandelier National Monument, Jemez State Monument, Chaco Canyon, and Gila Cliff Dwellings National Monument are just a few of the historic sites New Mexico offers. Due to constant attacks by nomadic bands of Apache, New Mexico was protected by 18 permanent forts and many more temporary cavalry camps. Six of the cavalry posts were home to Buffalo Soldiers.

Rock hounds keep busy in New Mexico year-round, attracted by quartz, turquoise, and dozens of other minerals. Many old mines dot the state and provide fascinating tales of wild and rowdy boomtowns that quickly became ghost towns as the gold and silver strikes played out. New Mexico is rich in history. If you love the Old West, we have a wild and wooly experience waiting for you. Dozens of crumbling ghost towns await your discovery. Fort Sumner is the final resting place of Billy the Kid. West of Ruidoso, New Mexico, you'll find the site of the Lincoln County Wars and the home and grave of Smokey Bear. New Mexico has two Civil War battlefields: Glorieta Pass and Valverde. Visit the historic border town of Columbus and retrace the steps of Pancho Villa's army as they perpetrated the famous raid in 1916.

New Mexico has the largest American Indian population in the nation, with more than 134,000 people. Twenty-two different tribal lands provide many diverse camping, hunting, fishing, hiking, and other recreational opportunities.

New Mexico is also the land of Spanish conquistadors. You can walk the same paths as Coronado, Sanchez, Chamuscado, Rodriguez, Gallegos, Espejo, Sosa, and de Onate as they went searching for the treasures of the seven cities of Cibola.

Numerous cattle trails also await your exploration. If you're a railroad buff, the rich history of the Atchison, Topeka, and Santa Fe Railroad expansion of the 1800s might interest you. You can camp near the birthplace of the great Apache warrior Geronimo in the Gila River Valley and explore the same trails and hideouts used by Geronimo, Cochise, Mangas Coloradas, and Victorio, who evaded capture for 25 years.

Hundreds of miles of equestrian trails offer the delight of a trail ride or camping on horseback. If you enjoy backcountry camping, check out the endless opportunities available to backpackers. Off-road motorcycle and all-terrain-vehicle trails lead to remote wild country where few venture, but be sure to check the laws regarding off-road vehicle use before heading out.

New Mexico is a land of deep forests, every bit as lovely as the other Rocky Mountain states. Because the Southern Rockies are generally more arid than the mountain states to the north, New Mexico is susceptible to extreme fire danger. During dry periods, the forests can become a lethal tinderbox in a short period of time. In the 1980s through the early 2000s, we experienced severe drought resulting in forest closures. When we experience a dry spell, be prepared to camp without a campfire. Stage II restrictions (no campfires) may go into effect with little warning, but campstoves are still allowed. Camping during Stage II fire restrictions is a delightful experience because the campgrounds are less crowded and the fragrances of the forests are indescribable.

So, *bienvenidos!* Welcome to New Mexico!

## :: WEATHER

Because of its southerly location, New Mexico has a climate that attracts scores of outdoor enthusiasts. Springtime comes earlier than it does for our neighbors to the north, and fall remains longer. For the "fair weather" outdoors enthusiast, this means the camping season can begin as early as March and extend well into November. Many campgrounds open as early as March to accommodate spring turkey hunts and remain open late for elk and deer hunting. Campers begin their treks in early spring in the lowland desert, moving to the higher elevations as the weather warms, then return to the lower elevations in late fall.

Spring is the most variable season. During March you'll find your first signs of rebirth in the lowlands, yet trees in the high country reach full foliage by late May to early June. Both winter- and summerlike weather can occur in spring. New Mexico is notoriously windy in the spring and the fall, so be prepared. Through mid-May, the high country can experience daytime temperatures of 60°F and nighttime temperatures that drop below freezing. Be prepared for cold fronts—temperatures can rapidly drop, and cold-weather apparel is a must. Keep an eye on the forecast and pack warm sleeping bags. New Mexico's spring weather is usually dry, and Stage II fire restrictions (no campfires allowed) are common.

Desert campgrounds in the lowlands are ideal locations to begin the camping season, with daytime temperatures in the 60–70°F range and nighttime temperatures in the 40–50°F range. This is the ideal time to experience the Chihuahuan Desert. Many southern New Mexico campgrounds have cactus and succulent gardens, which begin blooming in March and continue to do so through the month of May. Desert yucca blooms at the same time, with incredible white blossoms bending in the warm breezes. Sage begins growing at the same time, painting the desert floors a silvery green.

Summers begin in mid-May in the high country. June temperatures can soar into the 80°F range but rarely go higher. Nights are usually cool and can drop into the mid-40s at elevations of 8,000 feet or more. Summer sunrises and sunsets are incredible, with clouds on the horizon; majestic pinks, fiery reds, and yellows paint New Mexico skies with indescribable beauty. As July approaches, the monsoon season arrives, dousing the thirsty mountains with much-needed rain. The rains bring cold fronts, and temperatures that plummet into the 40–50°F range are common. Precipitation levels have increased significantly in the last decade, bringing rain on an almost daily basis to many areas, so pack rain gear and have a tarp handy for the picnic table. Our desert campgrounds are delightful when the monsoon season arrives—hiking in the warm summer rain is a wonderful experience.

Lowland-desert camping in summer can be challenging, and temperatures in excess of 100°F are common. The lakes and rivers throughout the state are popular and become quite

# Life Zones of New Mexico

## LOWER SONORAN
### To 4,500 feet
- Temperature and evaporation high, precipitation low
- Characteristic plants: Mesquite, creosote, greasewood, yucca, agave, four wing saltbrush, native grasses
- Characteristic animals: Coatamundi, javelina, ringtail cat, desert bighorn sheep, coyote, mountain lion, rattlesnake, lizard, box turtle

## UPPER SONORAN
### 4,500-7,500 feet
- Temperature modest to high, evaporation high, precipitation modest
- Characteristic plants: Alligator juniper, Chihuahua pine, chamisa, cholla, Apache plume, Gambel oak, box elder, salt cedar, cottonwood, pinon, juniper, red cedar
- Characteristic animals: White-tailed deer, mule deer, pronghorn antelope, black bear, prairie dog, rabbit

## TRANSITION
### 7,500 feet-8,200 feet
- Milder summer, cold winter, substantial rain and snow, evaporation modest
- Characteristic plants: Ponderosa, limber, and Apache pine; mountain maple; New Mexico locust; river willow
- Characteristic animals: Elk, beaver, bobcat, fox, Abert's squirrel

## NORTHERN CONIFEROUS FOREST
### 8,200 feet-10,000 feet
- Cool summers, cold winters, high amounts of rain and snow, evaporation modest to low
- Characteristic plants: Douglas fir, white fir, spruce, blue spruce, alpine juniper, limber pine, bristlecone pine, aspen
- Characteristic animals: High populations of elk, Rocky Mountain bighorn sheep, mountain marmot

## ALPINE TIMBERLINE AND ABOVE
### 10,000 feet and up
(Timberline varies in elevation depending upon latitude and slope.)
- Temperatures cool to cold, high amounts of rain and snow, high evaporation, high wind, high exposure, severe weather possible year-round
- Characteristic plants: Low hardy grasses, dwarf shrubs and sedges, algae, lichens
- Characteristic animals: High populations of elk and Rocky Mountain bighorn sheep

crowded. Sunscreen and polarized sunglasses are essential; the New Mexico sun is bright. Sunstroke is a constant danger, so take precautions and stay hydrated. Shade is a priority, but campgrounds with adequate shade trees are uncommon in the desert, so a shade shelter is a wise investment.

In the high country the monsoon season often means extreme danger. Often, the Forest Service will close certain recreation areas near forest fire burn scars. Flash floods occur when rain flows down steep mountainsides that have burned. The remaining burn scar areas can no longer maintain the deluge, and the rain races down mountainsides, creating extreme flash flooding.

Autumn arrives in the high country in mid-September, and most campgrounds close by October, with the exception of campgrounds near popular hunting areas. U.S. Forest Service campgrounds may lock some loops because of dwindling crowds. Fall usually sees an increase of activity in the lowlands, with the warm autumn days hovering around 70–80°F until November. Evening temperatures in the lowlands rarely drop below 40°F through November.

The first snows of winter usually arrive in the higher elevations in November, and snow can continue through April. Annual winter snowfall can vary from 40 to 120 inches. Expect to incur entire days of below-freezing weather; temperatures may range from mild to bitterly cold. High-country campgrounds usually close at the first signs of snow and open after the snow has melted. A few state park campgrounds remain open. Always call ahead for campground-closure information.

The lowland-desert campgrounds in the southern parts of New Mexico become quite busy in the winter. Snowbirds arrive in November and stay until March, fueling the economies of many communities with much-needed revenue. Winter tent camping is delightful in the deserts, with daytime temperatures in the 50–60°F range and nights in the 30–40°F range.

## :: FIRST-AID KIT

A useful first-aid kit may contain more items than you might think necessary. These are just the basics. Prepackaged kits in waterproof bags (Atwater Carey and Adventure Medical make them) are available. As a preventive measure, take along sunscreen and insect repellent. Even though quite a few items are listed here, they pack down into a small space:

- Ace bandages or Spenco joint wraps

- Adhesive bandages, such as Band-Aids

- Antibiotic ointment (Neosporin or the generic equivalent)

- Antiseptic or disinfectant, such as Betadine or hydrogen peroxide

- Aspirin, acetaminophen, or ibuprofen

- Benadryl or the generic equivalent, diphenhydramine (in case of allergic reactions)

- Butterfly-closure bandages

- Comb and tweezers (for removing ticks from your skin)

- Dark chocolate (won't cure anything, but it'll sure make you feel better)

- Epinephrine in a prefilled syringe (for severe allergic reactions to such things as bee stings)

- Gauze (one roll and six 4-by-4-inch compress pads)

- LED flashlight or headlamp

- Matches or lighter

- Moist towelettes

- Moleskin/Spenco 2nd Skin

- Pocketknife or multipurpose tool

- Waterproof first-aid tape

- Whistle (it's more effective in signaling rescuers than your voice)

## :: ANIMAL HAZARDS

### Black Bears

New Mexico has one species of bear, the North American black bear (*Ursus americanus*). Black bears are not an endangered species, and it is estimated that up to 5,000 bears reside in New Mexico with a population of over 900,000 in North America. Campgrounds at more than 5,000 feet elevation in New Mexico are in bear country. Since 2000, 14 deaths have been linked to black-bear attacks. There have been 56 documented human deaths by black bears in North America in the past 100 years. Black bears generally attack humans only when provoked or startled.

### Facts about Black Bears

- Black bears are the most common species of bear in North America.
- Adult male bears weigh up to 600 pounds; female bears weigh up to 400 pounds.
- Standing up on its hind feet, a black bear can tower up to 7 feet tall.
- Although black bears generally have shaggy black hair, the coat can vary in color from white to chocolate brown, cinnamon brown, and blonde. They occasionally have a slight V-shaped white chest blaze.
- Black bears have a large range that can encompass hundreds of square miles.
- Black bears can run over 30 miles per hour, are adept at climbing trees, and are excellent swimmers.
- Black bears rarely make false charges to intimidate; if the bear lunges, it will attack.

- Black bears hunt and forage mostly at night and are less active during the day.
- Black bears see in color and their vision is equal to that of a human; night vision is far superior.
- Black bears' hearing exceeds human frequency ranges and is estimated at twice the sensitivity.
- Black bears have a keen sense of smell, estimated at 500 times the sensitivity of a human. Bears have an ability to detect food up to a distance of 10 miles.
- Black bears can live up to 33 years.

## Bear-proofing Your Camp

- Consult with rangers, camp hosts, and other campers regarding recent bear sightings.
- Abide by all posted warning signs and bulletins posted by the ranger office.
- Keep all food stored in your vehicle or animal-proof storage lockers between meals and when leaving the campsite, even for short periods of time.
- Stow cookware, all spices, and hummingbird feeders, both while away from camp and overnight, inside a vehicle or animal-proof storage lockers.
- Keep a clean camp; throw trash away frequently.
- Never throw any food items in the campfire.
- Never take any foods or drinks inside tents.
- Store any clothing that was worn while preparing food or eating a meal inside a vehicle.
- Keep pets on leashes at all times. Pets are a very good early-warning alarm when bears are near.
- Dispose of unfinished beer and sugary drinks away from your camp.

## If a Bear Enters Your Camp

- Do not panic and do not run; gather all members of your party and your pets, and quietly get in your vehicle. (Keep car doors unlocked during the day while in camp for quick entry.)
- Make every attempt to avoid confronting the bear if possible. Use bear repellent only; do not use pepper spray meant for humans or dogs.
- Use whistles or car panic alarms in an attempt to scare the bear away.
- As a last resort, kill an attacking bear; use a weapon of no less than .38 caliber. A warning shot may not stop a charge.

## *Venomous Snakes*

All venomous snakes in New Mexico are very dangerous and should be avoided at all costs. Snakes can be upset by human presence and can unexpectedly become aggressive. Do not

give them a reason or an opportunity to attack. Always keep your distance. Your safety is your responsibility.

Familiarize yourself with the snakes of the area you are traveling into, both venomous and nonvenomous species. Reptile guidebooks are beneficial for identification, but the best way to prevent a snakebite is to steer clear of all snakes. Learn which habitats the venomous species in your region are likely to be encountered in, and use caution when in those habitats. Always take a buddy into the field with you; do not hike alone. Wear ankle-high boots and loose-fitting pants.

Make noise on the trail to avoid surprising snakes. Stay on trails, and watch where you place your hands and feet, especially when climbing or stepping over fences, large rocks, and logs, or when collecting firewood. At the campground, tread cautiously around rock outcroppings and downed trees.

Of the 8,000 snakebite victims in the United States each year, only about 10 to 15 die. However, for any snakebite, the best course of action is to get medical care as soon as possible.

- Keep the snakebite victim still, as movement helps the venom spread through the body.
- Keep the injured body part motionless and just below heart level.
- Keep the victim warm, calm, and at rest, and transport the victim immediately to medical care. Do not allow victim to eat or drink anything.
- If medical care is more than half an hour away, wrap a bandage a few inches above the bite, keeping it loose enough to enable blood flow (you should be able to fit a finger beneath it). Do not cut off blood flow with a tight tourniquet. Leave the bandage in place until reaching medical care.
- If you have a snakebite kit, wash the bite and place the kit's suction device over the bite. (Do not suck the poison out with your mouth.) Do not remove the suction device until you reach a medical facility.
- Try to identify the snake so that the proper antivenin can be administered, but do not waste time or endanger yourself trying to capture or kill it.
- If you are alone and on foot, start walking slowly toward help, exerting the injured area as little as possible. If you run or if the bite has delivered a large amount of venom, you may collapse, but a snakebite seldom results in death.

The five most common venomous snakes in New Mexico are the timber rattlesnake, Western diamondback rattlesnake, sidewinder rattlesnake, speckled rattlesnake, and Western coral snake. The four rattlesnake species belong to the pit-viper family, and the coral snake belongs to the cobra family. The fangs of the cobra-snake family are fixed in place and do not fold back inside the lower jaw as do pit-viper fangs.

**Timber Rattlesnake** (*Crotalus horridus*) 35–74" Colors of snake range from yellowish-, brownish- or pinkish-gray, with tan or reddish-brown back stripe dividing chevronlike cross bands. There are dark stripes behind the eyes. Timber rattlesnakes are active from April to October in the daytime in spring and fall and at night in summer. Timber rattlesnakes congregate in large numbers about rocky den sites. They are often encountered coiled up waiting for prey (squirrels, mice, chipmunks, small birds); if you see one, remain motionless. Record longevity exceeds 30 years. Timber rattlesnakes make their abode in elevations of more than 6,600 feet and are the most common rattlesnake species found in the high elevations of New Mexico.

**Western Diamondback Rattlesnake** (*Crotalus atrox*) 34–83" This is the largest Western rattlesnake. The snake is heavy bodied with large head sharply distinct from neck. The back is patterned with light-bordered dark diamonds or hexagonal blotches. There are two light diagonal lines on each side of its face. A stripe behind the eye meets the upper lip well in front of the angle of the jaw. The snake's tail is encircled by broad black-and-white rings. Known as the coon tail rattler, this dangerous reptile is most active late in the day and at night during hot summer months, but can be seen from April through October. It eats rodents and birds. Record longevity is nearly 26 years. When disturbed it stands its ground, lifts its head well above its coils, and sounds a buzzing warning. Its habitat is in arid and semiarid areas from plains to mountains: brushy desert, rocky canyons, bluffs along rivers, and sparsely vegetated rocky foothills; it is found from sea level to 7,000 feet in elevation.

**Sidewinder** (*Crotalus cerastes*) 17–32" The sidewinder is a rough-scaled rattler with a prominent triangular, hornlike projection over each eye. It travels over surfaces by "sidewinding." It leaves a trail of parallel J-shaped markings. Primarily nocturnal, it is usually encountered crossing roads between sundown and midnight in spring. During the day it occupies mammal burrows or hides in shelters beneath bushes. The sidewinder eats pocket mice, kangaroo rats, and lizards. This snake is active from April to October, late in the day and at night during hot summer months. This snake predominately prefers arid desert flatland and sandy arroyos, and is found up to 5,000 feet in elevation.

**Speckled Rattlesnake** (*Crotalus mitchellii*) 23–52" This rattlesnake's pattern and color vary greatly; it is most commonly seen with a sandy, speckled appearance. The rattlesnake is active during the day in spring and fall, at night in summer. It eats ground squirrels, kangaroo rats, white-footed mice, birds, and lizards. Record longevity exceeds 16 years. The rattlesnake prefers rugged rocky terrain, rock outcrops, deep canyons, taluses, chaparral amid rock piles and boulders, and rocky foothills up to 8,000 feet in elevation.

**Western Coral Snake** (*Micruroides euryxanthus*) 13–21" The Western coral snake is blunt-snouted and glossy, with alternating wide red, wide black, and narrow yellow or white rings encircling the body. The head is uniformly black to the angle of the jaw; its scales are smooth. This snake emerges at night, usually during or following a warm shower. When disturbed, it buries its head in its coils, raises and exposes the underside of its tail, and may make a popping sound. This snake is the most dangerous snake in New Mexico, and its venom is highly toxic. The Western coral snake eats blind snakes or other small snakes. It prefers rocky areas, plains to lower mountain slopes, and rocky upland desert—especially in arroyos and river bottoms up to 5,900 feet in elevation.

## Scorpions and Centipedes

Scorpions have long been of interest to humans primarily because of their ability to give painful and sometimes life-threatening stings. Scorpions are venomous arthropods in the class Arachnida, relatives of spiders, mites, ticks, and others. Scorpions have an elongated body and a segmented tail that is tipped with a venomous stinger. They have four pairs of legs and plierlike pincers, which are used for grasping. The species include:

**Desert Grassland Scorpion** (*Paruroctonus utahensis*) The desert grassland scorpion spends most of its reclusive life in its burrow to minimize exposure to predation. The venom of this scorpion results in a painful sting, but it's rarely fatal unless an allergic reaction occurs. This species of scorpion resides in shifting sands in the Mexican state of Chihuahua, and in Arizona, New Mexico, Texas, and Utah. This scorpion is pale yellow to yellowish-brown matching local sand color. Pincers are swollen and keeled with short fingers in adults. Legs have bristle combs that provide traction on sandy ground. An obligate burrower, it often digs its burrow at the base of vegetation on sand dunes. This species potentially lives six to seven years.

**Desert Hairy Scorpion** (*Hadrurus arizonensis*) The desert hairy scorpion is the largest scorpion in North America, obtaining a length of up to 6 inches. Their bodies are brown, with yellowish pincers and legs. Their common name comes from the brown hairs that cover their bodies. It is not dangerous to humans unless an allergic reaction occurs. This species is aggressive, though, and will sting readily. The desert hairy scorpion gets its water from the animals it feeds on. This has proven to be a popular scorpion species in captivity due to its size, beauty, and low risk of danger.

**Arizona Bark Scorpion** (*Centruroides sculpturatus*) This species is universally tan and grows to a length of 2½ inches; it is the most commonly encountered house scorpion. The Arizona bark scorpion is the only species in North America with venom potent enough to be dangerous to humans. The sting of this scorpion can be fatal to humans, particularly to infants and small children, so it is important to be careful when picking up firewood or rocks. Although the sting of this scorpion has killed more people in Arizona than all types of poisonous snakes combined, not one documented death has occurred in the United States for more than 30 years.

**Giant Redheaded Centipede** (*Scolopendra heros*) Centipedes, named for the erroneous belief that they have 100 feet, rarely have more than 60 or 70 feet. These centipedes attract a great deal of attention because of their fierce appearance and size, growing up to 8 inches long.

The centipede's bite is followed by a sharp and strictly local pain that subsides after about 15 minutes. In about two hours the pain is only very slight, but there is a general swelling in the bite location. Three hours after the bite, most symptoms will disappear. The bite of a typical centipede can be very painful for humans, similar to that of a wasp sting, and can usually be treated with an antihistamine if no infection develops. Centipede bites to children and those who are allergic require prompt medical attention.

## *Other Animal Threats*

Coyotes and foxes generally don't frequent campgrounds, but they are shrewd predators and will snatch unattended pets. Mountain lions and bobcats are rarely sighted, but be wary. Utilizing bear-proofing methods ensures these predators will not be as likely to invade your camp. Mexican gray wolves were controversially reintroduced in the Gila Mountains in the 1990s; they are successfully breeding in the Gila. All warm-blooded animals can carry rabies, so be careful.

Rodents can get into food, so keep everything packed away when you aren't cooking. Raccoons can wreak havoc at your campground. Hantavirus, plague, and other diseases are carried by campground rodents.

By all means, keep your tent zipped shut at all times when camping in New Mexico. Mosquitoes aren't quite as common as in many other states due to the arid climate. Bees and wasps are most common around rivers and lakes. Be prepared for encounters with snakes, scorpions, and centipedes. Don't leave your footwear outside of the tent, and make a habit of shaking out your shoes and boots prior to putting them on.

### :: PERMITS AND PASSES

The National Park Service offers a series of America the Beautiful passes, which can be used at all federal campgrounds and parks operated by the National Park Service, U.S. Forest Service, Bureau of Land Management, and U.S. Army Corps of Engineers. The annual pass costs $80 and is available to everyone (annual passes are free to all military members and their dependents); the senior pass is $10 for a lifetime pass and is available to US citizens and permanent residents age 62 and older; the access pass is free to US citizens and permanent residents with permanent disabilities. These passes can be obtained at any federal recreation site. For a list of these sites and more information on these passes, visit **nps.gov.** Passes must be in full view on your windshield or dash for the duration of your stay. Note that Golden Access and Golden Age Passports are no longer sold but continue to be honored.

If you make a reservation through **reserveamerica.com** or **recreation.gov,** the above passes entitle you to a 50% discount for the campsite that your access pass provides. You must provide the number from your placard or pass card when you reserve the campsite. You must still pay the full service charge for making the reservation, and all service fees from the reserveamerica.com or recreation.gov reservation system will apply. Please refer to the website for current service charges.

New Mexico state parks *do not* honor the America the Beautiful passes, but the following annual camping permits are available for New Mexico state parks: $180 New Mexico resident, $100 senior New Mexico resident (age 62 and older), $100 disabled New Mexico resident, and $225 nonresident. For more information, visit **www.emnrd.state.nm.us.**

### :: FIRE SAFETY

It is mandatory to carry a shovel and axe (or hatchet) when you camp in New Mexico. When tent camping, carry a lawn rake as well and rake a large radius free of combustibles from around the fire ring. Please use only water to douse your campfire; do not use dirt. Discard cold ashes in trash bags, not under trees or in streams. *Note:* It is imperative that you familiarize yourself with the fire restrictions for New Mexico before you go camping. These can be found at **firerestrictions.us/nm.** Also visit **nmfireinfo.com** for additional information on keeping our forests safe.

## :: HAPPY CAMPING

There is nothing worse than a bad camping trip, especially because it is so easy to have a great time. To assist with making your outing a happy one, here are some pointers.

- Reserve your site in advance, especially if it's a weekend or a holiday, or if the campground is wildly popular. Many prime campgrounds require at least a six-month lead time on reservations. Check before you go.

- Also, because of state and federal budget restrictions, campground management may limit recreational opportunities. This is another good reason to always call ahead for the current status of any campground in this guide.

- Pick your camping buddies wisely. A family trip is pretty straightforward, but you may want to reconsider including grumpy Uncle Fred, who doesn't like bugs, sunshine, or marshmallows. After you know who's going, make sure that everyone is on the same page regarding expectations of difficulty (amenities or the lack thereof, physical exertion, and so on), sleeping arrangements, and food requirements.

- Don't duplicate equipment, such as cooking pots and lanterns, among campers in your party. Carry what you need to have a good time, but don't turn the trip into a cross-country moving experience.

- Dress for the season. Educate yourself on the temperature highs and lows of the specific part of the state you plan to visit. It may be warm at night in the summer in your backyard, but up in the mountains it will be quite chilly.

- Pitch your tent on a level surface, preferably one covered with leaves, pine straw, or grass. Use a tarp or specially designed footprint to thwart ground moisture and to protect the tent floor. Do a little site maintenance, such as picking up the small rocks and sticks that can damage your tent floor and make sleep uncomfortable. If you have a separate tent rainfly but don't think you'll need it, keep it rolled up at the base of the tent in case it starts raining at midnight.

- Camping in New Mexico, you will find nice grassy forest floors are the exception rather than the rule. Rocky soil and hard-packed caliche clay are common. Consider taking a ground pad. When investing in a pad, shop for good quality. The best ground pads are self-inflating, with adequate foam padding inside. Avoid using inflatable air mattresses, which conduct heat away from the body and tend to deflate during the night.

- If you are not hiking in to a primitive campsite, there is no real need to skimp on food due to weight. Plan tasty meals and bring everything you will need to prepare, cook, eat, and clean up.

■ If you decide to bring water jugs to fill at the campground, take precautions to ensure water purity. I use the TastePURE brand water filter from Camco Manufacturing. It is an inline filter for RVs and lasts tent campers several years. Every campground treats well water with chlorine to kill bacteria, which may be noticeable in the smell and taste. Therefore, filtering is universally recommended.

■ If you tend to use the bathroom multiple times at night, you should plan ahead. Leaving a warm sleeping bag and stumbling around in the dark to find the restroom—whether it be a pit toilet, a fully plumbed comfort station, or just the woods—is not fun. Keep a flashlight and any other accoutrements you may need by the tent door and know exactly where to head in the dark.

■ Standing dead trees and storm-damaged living trees can pose a real hazard to tent campers (foresters call these widow-makers for obvious reasons). These trees may have loose or broken limbs that could fall at any time. When choosing a campsite or even just a spot to rest during a hike, look up.

## :: CAMPING ETIQUETTE

Here are a few tips on how to create good vibes with fellow campers and wildlife you encounter.

■ Obtain all permits and authorization as required. Make sure that you check in, pay your fee, and mark your site as directed. Don't make the mistake of grabbing a seemingly empty site that looks more appealing than your site. It could be reserved. If you're unhappy with the site you've selected, check with the campground host for other options.

■ Leave only footprints. Be sensitive to the ground beneath you. Place all garbage in designated receptacles or pack it out if none are available. No one likes to see the trash that someone else has left behind.

■ Never spook animals. It's common for animals to wander through campsites, where they may be accustomed to the presence of humans (and our food). An unannounced approach, a sudden movement, or a loud noise startles most animals. A surprised animal can be dangerous to you, to others, and to itself. Give them plenty of space.

■ Plan ahead. Know your equipment, your ability, and the area where you are camping—and prepare accordingly. Be self-sufficient at all times; carry necessary supplies for changes in weather or other conditions. A well-executed trip is a satisfaction to you and to others.

■ Be courteous to other campers, hikers, bikers, and anyone else you encounter.

■ Strictly follow the campground's rules regarding the building of fires. Never burn trash. Trash smoke smells horrible, and trash debris in a fire pit or grill is unsightly.

# Northern
# New Mexico

# 1

# Canjilon Lakes Campgrounds

*Meadows of wildflowers abound, including Indian paintbrush and columbine.*

**Canjilon (pronounced can-hee-loan)** Lakes is a beautiful and remote campground located several miles west of the tiny community of Canjilon, along the very bumpy Forest Service Road 129. Cars can make the trip driving slowly, but four-wheel-drive vehicles are recommended. Some areas on the road will slow you to 5–10 miles per hour. I towed a small pop-up here years ago and will never do it again. Road conditions may deteriorate during rainy weather. The washboard road deters most RVs from making the trip here, which makes these two campgrounds ideal for tent campers. Three cold-water lakes are located just 3 miles apart.

Lower Canjilon Lake Campground has 11 sites, and Middle Canjilon Lake Campground has 36 sites; sites vary in size and privacy. Most sites are shady throughout the day. Select your site with regard to water runoff, because some locations become a mud bog. Many of the sites are grassy and ideal for tent camping. These two campgrounds rarely fill to capacity.

The vault toilets are modern and very clean. There is no water here; you must bring your own. Be sure to come well supplied because the bumpy drive to town isn't something you want to do once you get settled in. The ranger station is 1 mile north of the town of Canjilon on FR 129.

Security is great at these campgrounds. There is no evidence of vandalism, and Forest Service officers frequently patrol the area, with an occasional visit by New Mexico Department of Game and Fish and the Rio Arriba County Sheriff's Department.

Upper Canjilon Lake has no campground but features several picnic tables and a vault toilet for picnics and fishing. Area fishing is excellent, primarily for rainbow, brook, and cutthroat trout. Fishing licenses and possession limits are checked here on a regular basis, so be prepared. (Note that there are two other campgrounds in the area: Canjilon Creek has 4 sites, and Trout Lakes has 11 sites. The latter is accessible only by four-wheel-drive vehicles. Neither campground is profiled in this book.)

The altitude here is among the highest of all of the campgrounds profiled in this book. Temperatures dip down into the 40°F range many nights, even in July, and daytime temperatures rarely exceed 80°F. It can snow here anytime during the camping season. The altitude is partly what makes Canjilon so lovely. There are many aspen groves, tall ponderosa pines, spruce trees, and firs, with scrub oaks near the lakes and creeks. Wildflowers abound, including Indian paintbrush and columbine. Outside the campgrounds

## :: Ratings

BEAUTY: ★ ★ ★ ★ ★
PRIVACY: ★ ★ ★
SPACIOUSNESS: ★ ★ ★ ★
QUIET: ★ ★ ★ ★
SECURITY: ★ ★ ★
CLEANLINESS: ★ ★ ★ ★

## :: Key Information

| | |
|---|---|
| **ADDRESS:** Carson National Forest, Canjilon Ranger District, P.O. Box 469, Canjilon, NM 87515 | **PARKING:** At site |
| **OPERATED BY:** U.S. Department of Agriculture | **FEE:** $5, plus $5 per extra vehicle |
| | **ELEVATION:** *Lower Campground* 9,850 feet; *Middle Campground* 9,830 feet |
| **CONTACT:** 575 684 2489; fax 575-684-2486; **www.fs.usda.gov/carson** | |
| | **RESTRICTIONS** |
| **OPEN:** End of May–Sept. 12 | ■ **Pets:** On 6-foot leash only; this is black bear country and also home to mountain lions, bobcats, and coyotes, so monitor pets closely. |
| **SITES:** *Lower Canjilon Lakes Campground* 11; *Middle Canjilon Lakes Campground* 36 | |
| **SITE AMENITIES:** Parking space, picnic table, fire ring | ■ **Fires:** In fire rings only; charcoal grills permitted; check with campground host, Forest Service office, and postings on camp bulletin board for restrictions. |
| **ASSIGNMENT:** First come, first served; no reservations | |
| | ■ **Alcohol:** At campsites only |
| **REGISTRATION:** Self-registration on-site | ■ **Other:** Quiet hours 10 p.m.–6 a.m.; 14-day stay limit |
| **FACILITIES:** Vault toilets; bring water | |

are open meadows with tall prairie grass waving in the cool mountain breezes.

You will see some aspen groves defoliated in this area. These trees died as a result of an infestation of Western tent caterpillars, with past drought conditions, and other diseases contributing to their demise. Western tent caterpillars are widespread throughout the forests of the Southwest: More than 35,800 acres have fallen victim in New Mexico alone.

You will see evidence of beaver along nearby Canjilon Creek. Raccoons are regular pests here as well. There are no bear-proof food lockers, so store all food items in your vehicle.

Several nearby hiking trails may tire you out quickly due to the altitude. Nearby Canjilon Mountain tops out at 10,913 feet; Red Hill just due west is 10,108 feet at its summit. This entire area averages more than 9,000 feet in elevation.

## :: Getting There

From the town of Canjilon, drive northeast 12 miles on FR 129, and Lower Canjilon Lake will be on the left side of the road. Middle Canjilon Lake is 1 mile farther.

**GPS COORDINATES**

**Lower Lakes**   N36° 33.027'   W106° 20.693'

**Middle Lakes**   N36° 33.328'   W106° 19.947'

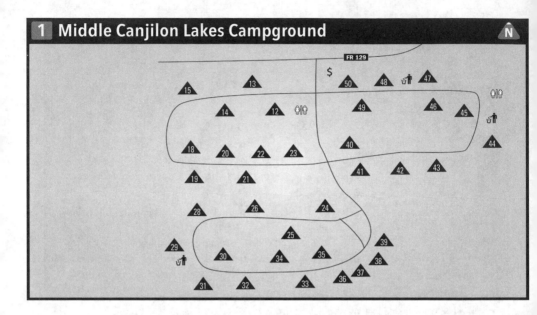

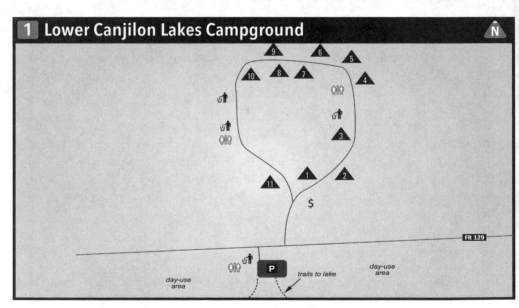

# 2

# Chaco Culture National Historical Park: GALLO CAMPGROUND

*You can hear the spirits of the old ones haunting the canyons.*

**H**ow would you like to camp within a few steps of ancient Anasazi cliff dwellings? If so, Chaco Culture National Historical Park is the place. Some say you can hear strange sounds at night—the spirits of the old ones haunting the canyons. I heard no spirits, just the rain spattering on my tent until way past midnight. I spent the evening reading all I could of the Anasazi culture that placed its indelible marks upon this beautiful canyon desert land.

Most New Mexico Pueblo Indian cultures hold this land sacred, so please be respectful and observe posted signs. The area is used by many tribes for religious ceremonies at different times of the year.

Chaco Canyon was a major Pueblo cultural center from AD 850 until 1250. The Pueblo Indians are known for architecture, astronomy, and artistry, and the visitor center has a museum with beautiful pottery displays and insight into the Anasazi way of life. A well-stocked bookstore with souvenirs supports the museum. A domed observatory for viewing the starry skies over

Chaco Canyon is free. Please inquire at the visitor center for operating times. Visitors are encouraged to bring their own telescopes. Several times a year different astronomy groups come to celebrate the incredible night skies with "star parties."

Past the visitor center are five ruins along a 9-mile circular loop, open from sunrise to sunset. The rockwork of the ruins is amazing, and the engineering and construction skills of the Anasazi are the real attraction at this location.

Mountain biking is allowed on certain trails with a free permit. Hiking the ruins is easy, but bring your camera, sunscreen, a hat, and water. Between the Pueblo Bonito ruins and the Chetro Ketl ruins is an amazing petroglyph trail, preserving 13 sites where pictographs can be seen and photographed. Interpretive booklets are available along the trail for a donation of 50 cents.

The campground is located off the right side of the paved access road 0.5 mile east of the visitor center. This is not a pretty campground. The ground is sandy; desert sage, tumbleweeds, and wild grasses intermingle with a few desert wildflowers. The beauty comes in the evening, when the pink and orange sunset paints the canyon walls and mesas with indescribable colors. The warm evening breezes cool many a weary hiker, and the coyote's song can be heard for miles. Several night birds provide melodies, and owls can be heard throughout the night.

## :: Ratings

BEAUTY: ★ ★ ★
PRIVACY: ★ ★ ★
SPACIOUSNESS: ★ ★ ★
QUIET: ★ ★ ★
SECURITY: ★ ★ ★ ★ ★
CLEANLINESS: ★ ★ ★ ★ ★

## :: Key Information

**ADDRESS:** Chaco Culture National Historical Park, P.O. Box 220, Nageezi, NM 87037

**OPERATED BY:** National Park Service

**CONTACT:** 505-786-7014 ext. 221; nps.gov/chcu

**OPEN:** Year-round 7 a.m.–sunset; visitor center open daily 8 a.m.–5 p.m. except Thanksgiving, Christmas, and New Year's Days, but the park's roads, sites, trails, and campground remain open.

**SITES:** 49, 2 group sites

**SITE AMENITIES:** Parking space, picnic table, gravel tent box, fire ring

**ASSIGNMENT:** Reserve at **recreation .gov;** 8 sites are first come, first served.

**REGISTRATION:** At visitor center

**FACILITIES:** Restroom, water spigot at visitor center

**PARKING:** At site

**FEE:** $15 individual site, $60 group site (10–30 people); individual entrance fee $4 for 7 days; vehicle entrance fee $8 for 7 days

**ELEVATION:** 6,215 feet

**RESTRICTIONS**

■ **Pets:** On 6-foot leash and under control at all times; allowed on backcountry hiking trails (on leash) but not within the archaeological sites; carry out all pet waste

■ **Fires:** In fire rings only; charcoal grills permitted; check with the visitor center or campground host for restrictions.

■ **Alcohol:** At campsites only

■ **Other:** Quiet hours 8 p.m.–8 a.m.; RV generators restricted to 1-hour intervals in campground; 14-day stay limit

The two modern restrooms are equipped with flush toilets and sinks. The restroom water supply is nonpotable; potable water is available at the visitor center. All sites are level. There's 1 accessible-only site, 15 tent-only sites, and 5 RV-only sites but no electric sites; most other sites are open to RVs or tents. Some sites are fully exposed with no shade whatsoever. It is wise to bring a sun shelter. Only a few sites are shaded by trees, and a few others are scattered among the boulders, which afford a little more shade and good privacy. But beware: These boulders are habitat for various species of rattlesnake.

Like most desert canyon campgrounds, Gallo is best enjoyed in the spring and fall when the weather is cooler. At this latitude and altitude, snows frequently blanket the area in winter, so come prepared.

From US 550, you will travel a 22-mile road; it's mostly dirt and can be muddy in spots. You have to cross an arroyo, which can flood with little warning; heed the signs. If the current is swift, do not tempt fate.

Bring everything you will need, as it's a 44-mile round-trip to US 550, which takes you to a convenience store called the Forty-Four Store with limited supplies. The town of Nageezi is a few miles north of the Forty-Four Store and has a trading post with groceries. Bring firewood; there is no firewood to gather inside the park.

## 2  Gallo Campground

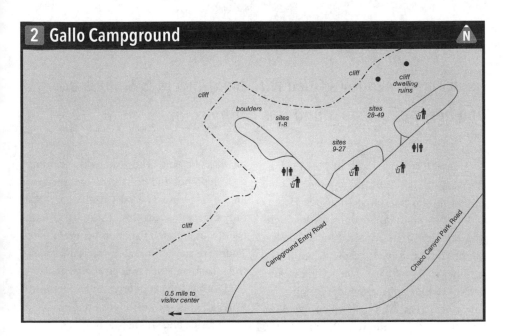

## :: Getting There

From Nageezi, take US 550 southeast 3 miles to CR 7900. Turn right onto CR 7900 (paved) and travel 8 miles. Take another right onto CR 7950 (a rough dirt road) and travel 13 miles to the park. The 4.5 miles before entering the park are very rough. Call the park at 505-786-7014 for current road conditions, and visit **nps.gov/chcu** for travel tips and more detailed directions.

**GPS COORDINATES**   N36° 1.940'   W107° 53.708'

# 3

# Hopewell Lake Campground

*Lush green meadows filled with wildflowers, grazing cattle, and herds of elk surround this campground.*

**L**ocated **20** miles west of Tres Piedras, Hopewell Lake lies along the 48-mile stretch of NM 64 connecting Tres Piedras and Tierra Amarilla. Sections of this highway are closed in winter. This is among the prettiest and most scenic drives in the nation. You'll enjoy views of rolling mountains with blue spruce, ponderosa pine, fir, and aspen trees. The lush green meadows are filled with wildflowers, grazing cattle, and occasionally herds of elk. This area is paradise for photographers.

You will see some aspen groves defoliated along NM 64. These trees died as a result of an infestation of Western tent caterpillars, with past drought conditions contributing to their demise. Western tent caterpillars are widespread throughout the forests of the Southwest: more than 35,800 acres have fallen victim in New Mexico alone. Despite the outbreak, the aspens within Hopewell Lake Campground are surviving nicely.

Hopewell Lake has two areas: the lake area and the campground. The lake area is for day use only. The road is quite bumpy as it descends the hill to the parking areas at the lakeside. The lake itself is small at only 25 water acres. It's stocked with rainbow trout, and the fishing is generally good. There are more than 20 picnic tables along the lakeshore, with a large shelter reserved for groups. Two modern vault toilets with water spigots and trash bins are provided at the lakeside and shelter.

Hopewell Lake Campground's one loop is quite large, with 32 campsites and four modern vault toilets. Trash bins and a water spigot are located at each toilet location. The well is deep and provides cold, sweet water. Most sites are large, well spaced, private, and very shady. However, sites 16, 17, 18, and 22 are in an open meadow and have no shade; sites 16 and 17 are reserved for equestrian campers. The ground is dirt, but there are many grassy areas for pitching tents. Sites 19–32 will appeal most to tent campers. RVs tend to prefer sites 1–15. The RV-to-tent ratio is about 50/50 at this campground, but with adequate distance between the sites, there is little interference. No generator-use restrictions exist at this campground. Campers will find plenty of firewood, mostly aspen, within the camp and in adjacent forest areas.

Trail riders and hikers have three different trails to explore. The trailheads are located across from site 10, between sites 15 and 16, and at a gated access road between

## :: Ratings

BEAUTY: ★ ★ ★ ★ ★
PRIVACY: ★ ★ ★ ★
SPACIOUSNESS: ★ ★ ★ ★
QUIET: ★ ★ ★ ★
SECURITY: ★ ★ ★
CLEANLINESS: ★ ★ ★ ★

## :: Key Information

**ADDRESS:** Carson National Forest, Tres Piedras Ranger District, P.O. Box 38, Tres Piedras, NM 87113

**OPERATED BY:** U.S. Department of Agriculture

**CONTACT:** 575-758-8678; www.fs.usda.gov/carson

**OPEN:** Mid-May–mid-Sept., weather permitting

**SITES:** 32

**SITE AMENITIES:** Parking space, picnic table, fire ring

**ASSIGNMENT:** Reserve at **reserve america.com** or **recreation.gov** or first come, first served.

**REGISTRATION:** Self-registration on-site without a reservation; with reservation, follow instructions on website and print receipt of reservation for check-in.

**FACILITIES:** Vault toilets

**PARKING:** At site

**FEE:** $15 individual site, $40 group area (plus $1 per person after 50 people)

**ELEVATION:** 9,850 feet

**RESTRICTIONS**

■ **Pets:** On 6-foot leash; take precautionary measures against predators.

■ **Fires:** In fire ring only; charcoal grills permitted; check with campground host, Forest Service office, and postings on camp bulletin board for restrictions.

■ **Alcohol:** At campsites only

■ **Other:** Quiet hours 10 p.m.–8 a.m.; 14-day stay limit

sites 16 and 17. The ruins of the old mining town of Hopewell, located to the west of the lake on the hillside, are also worth exploring.

Hopewell Lake Campground is less than 20 miles as the crow flies to the border of Colorado. The elevation is more than 9,800 feet high. Prepare for warm days in the 80s and cold nights in the 40s. Thunderstorms are common in this area, so be prepared to take shelter. Black bears, mountain lions, and bobcats are common; rein in the kids and pets.

The camp is patrolled by the Forest Service, and Rio Arriba County Sheriff Department officers may also make occasional stops at this camp. New Mexico game wardens check licenses and provide some security for the campground.

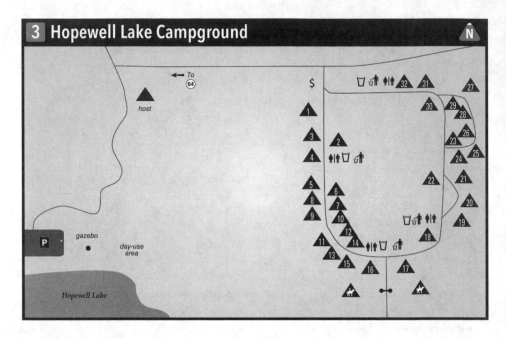

## :: Getting There

From Tres Piedras, drive west on NM 64 for 20 miles. You'll see the lake from the roadside, and there is a sign. Drive up the road past the lake entrance road, and the campground entrance is another 50 yards on the right.

**GPS COORDINATES**   N36° 42.092'   W106° 14.008'

# 4

# Columbine Campground

*Set along the Red River, Columbine is one of the loveliest campgrounds in New Mexico.*

**I**t is ironic that one of New Mexico's prettiest campgrounds sits right across the highway from one of the state's worst environmental disasters—the Molycorp Molybdenum Mine. The ugly mining scars will remain upon these mountains for thousands of years.

That said, the campground itself is still one of the loveliest in New Mexico. It sits in a dense growth of ponderosa pine, spruce, fir, aspen, and cottonwood. Tiny Columbine Creek runs through the campground, and if you select site 15, 17, 18, 26, or 27, you will be closest to this delightful meandering stream. There are four vault toilets, and several water spigots are available for potable water.

Columbine Creek flows into the Red River by the camp's entrance bridge. The river is stocked with trout from the nearby Red River Fish Hatchery, operated by the New Mexico Department of Game and Fish. It is an easy walk downhill to try your skill at fishing the river. New Mexico Game and Fish officers check for licenses and possession limits regularly.

## :: Ratings

BEAUTY: ★ ★ ★ ★ ★
PRIVACY: ★ ★ ★
SPACIOUSNESS: ★ ★ ★
QUIET: ★ ★ ★
SECURITY: ★ ★ ★ ★ ★
CLEANLINESS: ★ ★ ★ ★ ★

Columbine Campground is more grassy than the Red River campgrounds to the east (also profiled in this book), which is perfect for tent campers, but you can still expect a few RVs. It's also not as popular, which is a benefit for those who value privacy.

Campground traffic increases on weekends due to the Columbine Trailhead that begins in the camp. There is a separate parking area for hikers. The popular trail follows a gentle grade up Columbine Canyon and is rated easy to moderate. Access to the creek, wildflower-filled meadows, and occasional views of the high mountains to the south make this an ideal trail. Predators are common here, so watch children closely and keep your pets leashed.

The ice truck visits Columbine and delivers ice for the same price as at local stores. There is no firewood to gather at Columbine, but firewood is sold in the towns of Questa and Red River. Occasional firewood vendors stop by the camp to sell firewood at reasonable rates. Red River is 5.8 miles east, and Questa is 5.2 miles west of Columbine Campground. Red River is much more appealing to visit than Questa, but both towns offer full-service grocery stores, gas stations, and fishing and camping supplies.

In years past, no campground host has been assigned here, but plans are underway to assign one. The Forest Service, New Mexico Department of Game and Fish, and Taos

## :: Key Information

| | |
|---|---|
| **ADDRESS:** Carson National Forest, Questa Ranger District, 184 NM 38, Questa, NM 87556 | **PARKING:** At site |
| | **FEE:** $17, $5 per extra vehicle |
| **OPERATED BY:** U.S. Department of Agriculture | **ELEVATION:** 8,041 feet |
| **CONTACT:** 575-586-0520; www.fs.usda.gov/carson | **RESTRICTIONS** |
| | ■ **Pets:** On 6-foot leash; take precautionary measures against predators. |
| **OPEN:** May–Oct. 15, weather permitting | |
| **SITES:** 27 | ■ **Fires:** In fire rings only; charcoal grills permitted; check with campground host, Forest Service office, and postings on camp bulletin board for restrictions. |
| **SITE AMENITIES:** Parking space, picnic table, fire ring | |
| **ASSIGNMENT:** First come, first served | ■ **Alcohol:** At campsites only |
| **REGISTRATION:** Self-registration on-site | ■ **Other:** Quiet hours 10 p.m.–8 a.m.; 14-day stay limit |
| **FACILITIES:** Vault toilets | |

County Sheriff's Department frequently patrol this campground.

Because of the topography of the campground, road noise impacts Columbine Campground a little, but the campground sits back from the highway a bit. Because Columbine is nearly 800 feet lower in altitude, the weather is somewhat warmer than at the Red River camps. The snowfall here is less than at the Red River locations.

Nearby Goat Hill Campground is adjacent to NM 38 on the south side of the highway and isn't nearly as appealing as the other campgrounds nearby. The campground is shady but directly off the highway. The ground is crushed gravel and is better suited to trailers and small RVs than to tents. La Bobita Campground across the road would be much more appealing to campers than Goat Hill, but it's rarely open. If Columbine is full, you might try these camps as a backup.

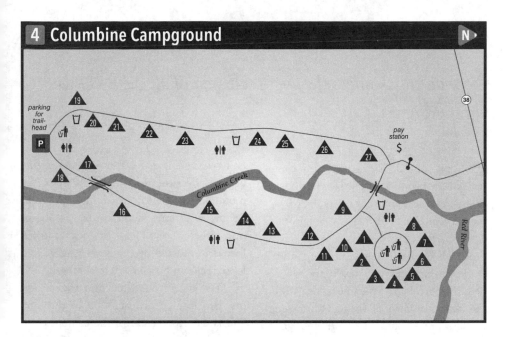

## :: Getting There

From Questa, turn east and follow NM 38 for 5.8 miles; turn right into the campground at the sign.

**GPS COORDINATES**   N36° 40.838'   W105° 30.918'

# 5

# Elephant Rock Campground

*Elephant Rock offers the best seclusion of all the Red River campgrounds.*

**S**et up on a hillside, this lovely campground is beautifully terraced with large campsites. Elephant Rock offers the privacy that Junebug or Fawn Lakes Campgrounds do not. This camp is often overlooked by those who prefer riverside camping and is the last campground nearest to the town of Red River to fill up on the weekends. It offers the best seclusion of all the Red River campgrounds. Most sites are large enough to accommodate two or more tents, and they're spaced a significant distance away from one another. You will see a few RVs here.

Elephant Rock Campground is across NM 38 from Fawn Lakes Campground; it's an easy 0.5-mile walk to Fawn Lakes. While driving down NM 38, watch closely for pedestrians, bicycles, and vehicles. Also look out for wildlife crossing the highway; it's busy during camping season.

The forest here is a mix of ponderosa pine, spruce, fir, and aspen trees. The hillside is rocky, but the large stone-terraced campsites are level and provide good water runoff. When it rains here, it can be a real gully washer. The views looking across the highway over the Red River Valley and the mountain range to the south are lovely. Behind this campground, the trees thin significantly to reveal Elephant Rock, at 10,556 feet. The hillside becomes very steep, and loose rock can be a hazard to climbers.

The campground has four water spigots, two located on each end of the loop and two in the center of the campground. The cold, sweet water is supplied from the city of Red River pumping station. There are three vault toilets, one at each end of the campground and one in the center. These facilities are extremely well maintained. In fact, the entire campground is very clean. The center of the campground provides kids with some running room, and the loop is fun for bicycling. Red River has excellent fishing; just walk across the highway.

There may be an occasional bear in the camp, but bears tend to spend more time along the river, across the highway. Mountain lions and bobcats can frequent this camp, so watch children closely and keep your pets leashed. You may also see the occasional mule deer.

The Forest Service, New Mexico state police, and the Taos County Sheriff's Department make regular patrols here—the security is very good. Campground hosts are also assigned here. Cellular service may be hit and miss at this location.

## :: Ratings

BEAUTY: ★ ★ ★ ★ ★
PRIVACY: ★ ★ ★ ★
SPACIOUSNESS: ★ ★ ★ ★
QUIET: ★ ★ ★ ★
SECURITY: ★ ★ ★ ★ ★
CLEANLINESS: ★ ★ ★ ★ ★

## :: Key Information

**ADDRESS:** Carson National Forest, Questa Ranger District, 184 NM 38, Questa, NM 87556

**OPERATED BY:** U.S. Department of Agriculture

**CONTACT:** 575-586-0520; www.fs.usda.gov/carson

**OPEN:** Weekend before Memorial Day–weekend after Labor Day

**SITES:** 22

**SITE AMENITIES:** Parking space, picnic table, fire ring

**ASSIGNMENT:** First come, first served

**REGISTRATION:** Self-registration on-site

**FACILITIES:** Vault toilets

**PARKING:** At site

**FEE:** $17, $5 per extra vehicle

**ELEVATION:** 8,440 feet

**RESTRICTIONS**

■ **Pets:** On 6-foot leash

■ **Fires:** In fire rings only; charcoal grills permitted; check with campground host, Forest Service office, and postings on camp bulletin board for restrictions

■ **Alcohol:** At campsites only

■ **Other:** Quiet hours 10 p.m.–8 a.m.; 14-day stay limit

As with all Red River campgrounds, the ice truck stops by regularly on weekends. The host usually sells firewood, and there are places to buy firewood at reasonable prices in Red River.

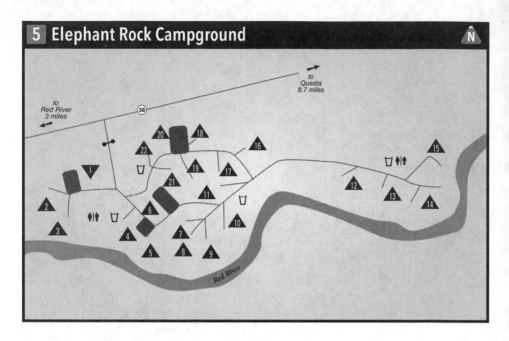

## :: Getting There

From Questa, turn east on NM 38 and drive 8.7 miles. Turn north into the campground.

**GPS COORDINATES**   N36° 42.352'   W105° 27.340'

# 6

# Fawn Lakes Campground

*Deeply entrenched in the Red River Valley, Fawn Lakes is encapsulated by mountains on both sides.*

**F**awn Lakes is a beautiful campground just 3.5 miles from the town of Red River. Like nearby Junebug Campground, it fills quickly most weekends. Fawn Lakes attracts RVs, but it is also ideal for tent camping. If you select a riverside campsite, you can pitch your tent close to the river for more privacy. The river can be heard throughout the campground and flows 25–50 cubic feet per second during the camping season. Watch small children carefully; the river water is cold and fast-flowing.

Fawn Lakes Campground sits deeply entrenched in the Red River Valley, encapsulated by mountains on both sides. In summer, daytime temperatures may reach 80°F. Evening temperatures drop quickly, so bring a warm jacket. Nighttime mercury may drop below 40°F, so bring warm sleeping bags.

Fawn Lakes is located right off NM 38, so some traffic noise can be heard at the sites close to the highway. If you camp near the river, you will never hear it. Fawn Lakes is very shady, with spruce, fir, ponderosa pine, aspen, cottonwood, and river willow

trees. Fishing is exceptional here; the river is stocked regularly by the Red River Hatchery, located 8 miles southwest of Questa.

Riverside campsites are spacious. Three tent sites are available off the end of the loop. There are two toilets, one located at the entrance and one located near the loop. Fawn Lakes has three water spigots, one at each end of the loop and the other at the center of the loop. The entire campground is very clean.

This is black bear country, so abide by the posted bear alerts, and you should be safe. Raccoons can be heard every night, so lock food in your vehicle. There are no bear-proof food lockers provided here. Broadtailed hummingbirds (*Selasphorus platycercus*) and rufous hummingbirds (*Selasphorus rufus*) are residents at this campground. Put away your feeder at night, though, because it will attract bears.

There's a campground host assigned here, and the Forest Service, New Mexico Department of Game and Fish, and Taos County Sheriff's Department patrol frequently. Fishing license and possession checks are conducted often, so be prepared.

Kids love Fawn Lakes, and there is much to keep them busy here. The three ponds called Fawn Lakes are an easy walk west of the campground. It's fun to feed and photograph the ducks in the pond. The ponds also have hiking trails that are a blast on a mountain bike.

## :: Ratings

> BEAUTY: ★ ★ ★ ★
> PRIVACY: ★ ★
> SPACIOUSNESS: ★ ★ ★
> QUIET: ★ ★ ★
> SECURITY: ★ ★ ★ ★ ★
> CLEANLINESS: ★ ★ ★ ★ ★

## :: Key Information

**ADDRESS:** Carson National Forest, Questa Ranger District, 184 NM 38, Questa, NM 87556

**OPERATED BY:** U.S. Department of Agriculture

**CONTACT:** 575-586-0520; **www.fs.usda.gov/carson**

**OPEN:** May–Oct.

**SITES:** 18

**SITE AMENITIES:** Parking space, picnic table, fire ring

**ASSIGNMENT:** Sites 1, 3–6, 8, 9, 12, 13, 16, and 17 accommodate tents and RVs and can be reserved at **reserveamerica .com;** sites 2, 7, 10, 11, 14, 15, and 18 are tent-only and first come, first served.

**REGISTRATION:** Self-registration on-site without a reservation; with reservation, follow instructions on website and print receipt of reservation for check-in.

**FACILITIES:** Vault toilets

**PARKING:** At site

**FEE:** $17, $5 per extra vehicle

**ELEVATION:** 8,515 feet

**RESTRICTIONS**

■ **Pets:** On 6-foot leash; black bears, mountain lions, and bobcats frequent this camp, so watch pets and children closely.

■ **Fires:** In fire rings only; charcoal grills permitted; check with campground host, Forest Service office, and postings on camp bulletin board for restrictions.

■ **Alcohol:** At campsites only

■ **Other:** Quiet hours 10 p.m.–8 a.m.; 14-day stay limit

A truck comes by selling block and cube ice on weekends. A gentleman sells firewood from his truck on weekends, and the campground host sells firewood for $3 a bundle. Campers can also purchase firewood in the nearby town of Red River.

Red River is a fun town with numerous restaurants and stores. Several saloons serve food and offer live bands on the weekends. A few outfitters cater to campers and anglers. Der Markt Grocery is a full-service store, and prices are reasonable. Cellular service is available in Red River, and cell phones also work at Fawn Lakes Campground. Free wireless high-speed Internet service is available at the new conference center just behind the park on Main Street. Internet service is also free at the Chamber of Commerce building. Try Texas Red's Steakhouse for a buffalo burger or a steak.

Many activities abound throughout the Red River Valley. Jeeps and ATVs can be rented in town, and four-wheel-drive vehicle tours are available. Horseback riding is also available here. The Circle of Enchantment drive covers 85 miles and encompasses some of the prettiest vistas in the United States. Visit Taos, Taos Pueblo, and Taos Mountain Casino. The Vietnam Memorial near the town of Angel Fire is a must, and the town and lake of Eagle Nest and the ghost town of Elizabethtown have worthwhile attractions.

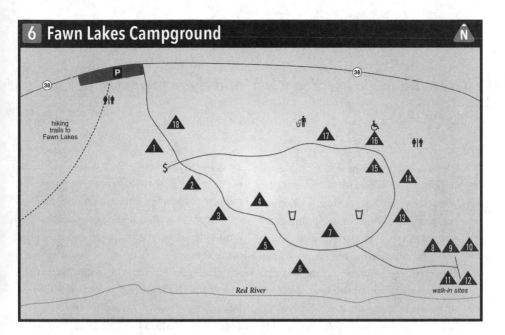

## :: Getting There

From Taos, go north on NM 522 to Questa. Turn east on NM 38 and travel 9.3 miles. The campground is on your right.

**GPS COORDINATES**   N36° 42.445'   W105° 26.958'

# 7

# Junebug Campground

*There is no place like Red River, and there is no campground like Junebug.*

**I**'ve been coming to Junebug since 1991. This pretty campground is just 2 miles from Red River and fills most weekends. Junebug gets a few RVs, but you'll find great tent camping here. Pick a spacious riverside campsite and pitch your tent close to the river. The river can be heard throughout the campground and flows between 25–50 cubic feet per second during the camping season. The Red River Valley is deeply entrenched by mountains on both sides. In the summer it rarely exceeds 80°F. When a cold front comes in, the temperature can drop rapidly, so bring a warm jacket. Nighttime temperatures may drop below 40°F, so pack warm sleeping bags too. Springtime is usually fairly dry, and Stage II fire restrictions may go into effect until July, when the monsoon season begins. But don't let that discourage you; come up and cold-camp. The forest has a lovely fragrance that is masked by wood smoke.

Junebug is very shady, with a mixture of spruce, fir, ponderosa pine, aspen, cottonwood, and river willow trees. Fishing is exceptional here; the river is stocked regularly by the Red River Hatchery, located 8 miles southwest of Questa. On our maiden trip here, our 8-year-old son caught our limit of trout before his mother and I got the camp set up.

The ground may be rocky in places, so bring a thick ground pad. There are two toilets, one located across from site 4 and another located on the end loop. The entire campground is very clean. Two water spigots serve Junebug, one at the entrance and another across from site 2. The water is icy cold and sweet and is Red River City Water.

This is serious black bear country, and bears are occasionally spotted in town. Abide by the posted bear alerts, and you should be fine. Mountain lions and bobcats won't venture this close to the town of Red River. Coyotes have been spotted across the river from the camp, though, so rein in your pets. Raccoons are quite common at Junebug, so store your food in your vehicle. Hummingbirds love this campground, so bring your feeder. The most common species here are the broad-tailed hummingbird (*Selasphorus platycercus*) and the rufous hummingbird (*Selasphorus rufus*). They provide all-day entertainment and are easy to photograph. Put away your feeder at night, however, because it will attract bears and raccoons.

There's a campground host assigned here, and the Forest Service patrols regularly, as do the New Mexico Department of

## :: Ratings

BEAUTY: ★ ★ ★ ★
PRIVACY: ★ ★
SPACIOUSNESS: ★ ★ ★ ★
QUIET: ★ ★
SECURITY: ★ ★ ★ ★ ★
CLEANLINESS: ★ ★ ★ ★ ★

## :: Key Information

**ADDRESS:** Carson National Forest, Questa Ranger District, 184 NM 38, Questa, NM 87556

**OPERATED BY:** U.S. Department of Agriculture

**CONTACT:** 575-586-0520; **www.fs.usda .gov/carson**

**OPEN:** May–Sept.

**SITES:** 20

**SITE AMENITIES:** Parking space, picnic table, fire ring

**ASSIGNMENT:** First come, first served

**REGISTRATION:** Self-registration on-site

**FACILITIES:** Vault toilets

**PARKING:** At site

**FEE:** $17, $5 per extra vehicle

**ELEVATION:** 8,559 feet

**RESTRICTIONS**

■ **Pets:** On 6-foot leash; take precautionary measures against predators.

■ **Fires:** In fire rings only; charcoal grills permitted; check with campground host, Forest Service office, and postings on camp bulletin board for restrictions.

■ **Alcohol:** At campsites only

■ **Other:** Quiet hours 10 p.m.–8 a.m.; 14-day stay limit

Game and Fish and the Taos County Sheriff's Department. Have your fishing license with you because license and possession checks are frequent here.

The Memorial Day Red River Motorcycle Rally attracts more than 10,000 motorcycle riders; the town is built for 2,000. If you are a tent-packing Harley rider, you'll enjoy this campground.

Privacy and quiet are hard to find on weekends, so try to plan weekday camping. Anglers inevitably pass near your riverside campsite, but overall the campers here are courteous and respectful.

Every weekend a vendor comes by to sell ice; another vendor sells firewood. The campground host also sells firewood, and there are several places to buy firewood at a reasonable price in Red River. There are no firewood gathering areas nearby.

Red River is a fun and friendly town, with an ice cream shop, restaurants, and shopping. Several stores cater to campers and anglers. Der Markt Grocery is a full-service grocery, and prices are reasonable. You can ride the chairlift to the top of the ski area. From there, hiking trails lead to the summit of New Mexico's highest mountain, Wheeler Peak. The Circle of Enchantment drive is 85 miles long and features the cultural town of Taos, the Taos Pueblo, Taos Casino, the Vietnam Memorial in the town of Angel Fire, the town and lake of Eagle Nest, and the ghost town of Elizabethtown.

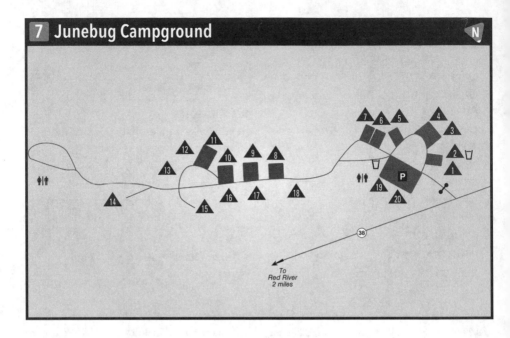

## :: Getting There

From Taos, go north on NM 522 to Questa. Turn east on NM 38 for 11 miles and turn into the campground on your right.

**GPS COORDINATES**  N36° 42.513'  W105° 26.222'

# 8

# Coyote Creek State Park

*This park explodes in color, with many varieties of wildflowers, oak trees, river willows, and ponderosa pines.*

**W**hen Louis L'Amour wrote his novel *The Sacketts,* he admitted his inability to describe the beauty of the Mora Valley. Words cannot do it justice. You have to experience it for yourself. Surrounded by ponderosa pine–covered mountains, this lush valley is filled with green pasturelands of cattle and horses grazing in the cool mountain breezes. The Mora Valley is old; dozens of crumbling adobe homes give testimony to the pioneers who tamed this majestic land. Several alpaca ranches in the area raise herds of these docile animals, and stores in the area sell alpaca wool products.

Coyote Creek State Park is 17 miles north of the town of Mora and is a premier tent-camper's park. Reserved RV campsites with full hookups are clustered together just past the comfort station, separating them from the rest of the park. All the other campsites are fairly well spread apart and are ideal for tent camping.

A large meadow runs the length of the park, filled with native grasses and abundant wildflowers. A modern playground in the meadow stays busy all day. Two campsites sit on top of the hill up a short dirt road. Both sites are equipped with an Adirondack shelter, as well as the standard picnic table and fire ring. Seven more campsites adjacent to the playground are large, well spaced, and private. Four of these seven sites are equipped with Adirondack shelters; the other three are under trees and shady. These sites can be used by either tents or RVs; they are reasonably level and grassy, making them ideal for tents.

The road continues through the meadow and across a bridge. Several sites are situated along the roadway, with shelters that will catch some dust. The RV dump station is located here. More tent sites are up the hill; these sites sit among oak, piñon, cedar, and ponderosa pine trees. The sites are dirt and have no grass, but they provide good tent camping with a great view. These sites are closer together, but private, due to the undergrowth of young trees and oak bushes.

Five modern vault toilets are distributed throughout the park and are kept very clean. The visitor center at the entrance is equipped with a spotless comfort station with sinks, flush toilets, and showers. The small office is open occasionally and stocks trail maps and state park information brochures.

One hiking trail circles the park, featuring footbridges, benches, an old moonshiner's shack, and a cold-water spring piped into a hewn-log livestock watering trough. The

## :: Ratings

BEAUTY: ★ ★ ★ ★ ★
PRIVACY: ★ ★ ★ ★
SPACIOUSNESS: ★ ★ ★ ★
QUIET: ★ ★ ★ ★ ★
SECURITY: ★ ★ ★ ★ ★
CLEANLINESS: ★ ★ ★ ★ ★

## :: Key Information

**ADDRESS:** Hwy. 434, Mile Marker 17, Guadalupita, NM 87722

**OPERATED BY:** New Mexico State Parks

**CONTACT:** 575-387-2328; **www.emnrd .state.nm.us/SPD/coyotecreeklakestate park.html**

**OPEN:** Year-round. In winter, water may not be available and park may be inaccessible; call ahead for details.

**SITES:** 47

**SITE AMENITIES:** Parking space, picnic table, fire ring; 4 sites equipped with Adirondack shelters

**ASSIGNMENT:** First come, first served or reserve at **reserveamerica.com** or 877-664-7787.

**REGISTRATION:** Self-registration on-site without a reservation; with reservation, follow instructions on website and print receipt of reservation for check-in.

**FACILITIES:** Restrooms, showers, vault toilets, visitor center, picnic shelter, playground

**PARKING:** At site

**FEE:** $8 primitive, $10 nonelectric, $14 with electric or sewage hookup, $18 with electric and sewage hookups; $5 day-use fee per vehicle

**ELEVATION:** 7,728 feet

**RESTRICTIONS**

■ **Pets:** On 10-foot leash; take precautionary measures against predators.

■ **Fires:** In fire rings only; charcoal grills permitted; check with campground host, Forest Service office, and postings on camp bulletin board for restrictions.

■ **Alcohol:** At campsites only; no glass permitted

■ **Other:** Quiet hours 10 p.m.–8 a.m.; 14-day stay limit

water from the spring is not potable. The trail is 1.5 miles and is more like a leisurely walk than a hike. Beware of nettles and poison ivy in the deep grass. The trail is alive with wildflowers from spring to fall, providing photographers with dozens of species. The park explodes in color in the fall, with oak trees and river willows providing the show, set among the ponderosa pine greenery.

For anglers, Coyote Creek is the most densely stocked water in New Mexico—12- to 15-inch rainbow trout are common. Within the park boundaries are two beaver ponds that provide excellent fishing spots along the stream. Coyote Creek is stocked with rainbow trout from the Mora Fish Hatchery every two weeks, and it is rated as one of the top fishing spots in the state.

Many birds are endemic to the park, and you can spot various raptors riding the air currents to the east over the mountain ridges. Black bears, mountain lions, bobcats, elk, mule deer, beavers, raccoons, skunks, and badgers make their homes in the surrounding mountains. Watch your children closely and be sure to keep your pets leashed. True to its name, this campground features free coyote concerts most nights, beginning just as you fall into a deep slumber. At night, the surrounding mountains are dimly silhouetted by the town lights of Mora to the south and Angel Fire to the north, yet the sky is pitch black and makes Coyote Creek a perfect place for stargazing.

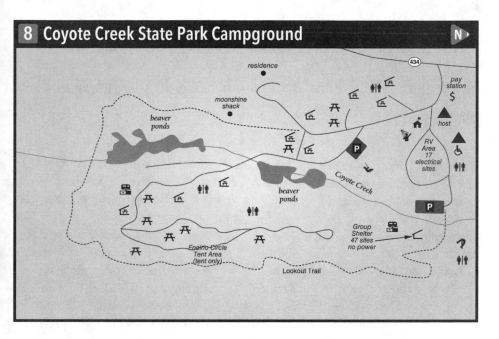

## 8 Coyote Creek State Park Campground

residence

moonshine
shack

beaver
ponds

434

pay
station

$

host

RV
Area
17
electrical
sites

P

Coyote Creek

beaver
ponds

Group
Shelter
47 sites
no power

P

Encino Circle
Tent Area
(tent only)

Lookout Trail

## :: Getting There

From Mora, New Mexico, turn right at the Coyote Creek State Park sign onto
NM 434 and travel 17 miles. The park turnoff is on the right.

**GPS COORDINATES**   N36° 10.680'   W105° 14.085'

# 9

# Morphy Lake State Park

*Shade is excellent here, provided by a healthy ponderosa pine forest.*

**B**eautiful **Morphy** Lake State Park is one of the best primitive tent-camping parks in New Mexico. Morphy Lake was accessible only by four-wheel drive for many years, but the road is now paved; however, it remains extremely steep in parts, with twists and turns, and is not for the faint of heart.

Morphy Lake is open year-round for ice fishing, but the campground is only open April 1 to November 1. Snow begins to fall as early as October, and winter storms are possible through late April. No snow removal is performed on this road. Off-season campers and anglers are encouraged to call ahead for road and weather conditions.

At the park entrance, a sign indicates trailers are limited to 18 feet due to tight turnarounds. Pop-up campers are common here. Little Morphy Lake is a pretty blue mountain lake with 15 water acres, and the park is just 30 land acres. Within its boundaries are 24 campsites circling the eastern, northern, and western sides of the lake. One hiking trail encircles the lake. Shade is excellent here, provided by a healthy ponderosa

pine forest. The campsites are considered developed, but there are no electric, water, or sewer hookups. Sites are not large, but each can accommodate any size tent, and most are fairly level and reasonably spaced apart. All sites have a spectacular view of the lake. Sites are dirt, with no grass, and because they're situated along the road, dust stirred up by cars or wind can be annoying.

To the west, views of 13,103-foot Trampas and 12,175-foot Truchas Peaks, as well as 12,500-foot Pecos Baldy, are spectacular. Snow is visible above timberline much of the year. It's best to take shoreline photos in the morning, with the peaks in the background.

Five clean vault toilets are equally spaced throughout the campground. There is no potable water here; you must bring in your own. There's also no firewood because the forest has been picked clean. Water and firewood are for sale in Mora, 11.5 miles away. Mora has several gas stations, a few cafés, a liquor store, and a full-service grocery with limited camping and picnic supplies.

Morphy Lake is great for canoes, kayaks, and inflatable boats, powered by paddle or electric trolling motors only. There is a concrete boat ramp. The lake is regularly stocked with trout from the Mora Fish Hatchery. A fishing tournament is held each August when the lake is filled with 600 20- to 22-inch rainbow trout.

Due to the park's remote location, predatory wildlife is common. You *must*

## :: Ratings

BEAUTY: ★ ★ ★ ★ ★
PRIVACY: ★ ★ ★
SPACIOUSNESS: ★ ★ ★
QUIET: ★ ★ ★ ★
SECURITY: ★ ★ ★ ★ ★
CLEANLINESS: ★ ★ ★ ★ ★

## :: Key Information

| | |
|---|---|
| **ADDRESS:** P.O. Box 477, Guadalupita, NM 87722 | **FEE:** $10 |
| **OPERATED BY:** New Mexico State Parks | **ELEVATION:** 8,057 feet |
| **CONTACT:** 575-387-2328; **www.emnrd .state.nm.us/SPD/morphylakestatepark .html** | **RESTRICTIONS**<br>■ **Pets:** On 10-foot leash; this is black bear country and also home to mountain lions, bobcats, coyotes, foxes, and badgers, so monitor pets closely. |
| **OPEN:** April 1–Nov. 1 | |
| **SITES:** 24 | ■ **Fires:** In fire rings only; charcoal grills permitted; check with campground host or New Mexico State Parks offices for restrictions. |
| **SITE AMENITIES:** Parking space, picnic table, fire ring | |
| **ASSIGNMENT:** First come, first served | |
| **REGISTRATION:** Self-registration on-site | ■ **Alcohol:** At campsites only; no glass permitted |
| **FACILITIES:** Vault toilets, boat ramp; bring water. | ■ **Other:** Quiet hours 10 p.m.–8 a.m.; 14-day stay limit; no refuse collection, so you must pack out your trash. |
| **PARKING:** At site | |

stow all food and trash in your vehicle at night; bear-proof storage boxes are not provided. Raccoons are common, too, and chipmunks scurry all over camp. Bring your hummingbird feeder because the little creatures are abundant. Elk, mule deer, skunks, badgers, black bears, mountain lions, bobcats, and coyotes reside in the forests nearby. A free coyote concert begins every morning between 3 and 5 a.m. Afternoon thunderstorms are common and can be potentially violent, with lightning.

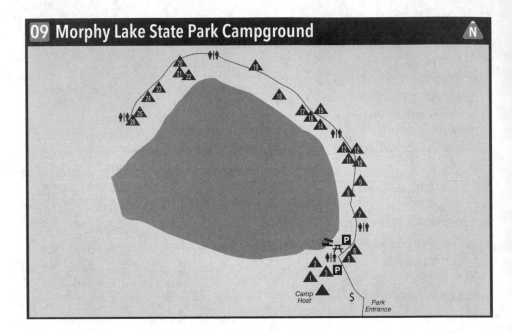

## :: Getting There

From Mora, head east on NM 518. Turn south onto NM 94 and travel 7 miles to the town of Ledoux. In Ledoux, turn right at the Morphy Lake sign onto Mora County Road 635, and drive 4 miles west. The road forks; take the right fork at the sign to the campground.

**GPS COORDINATES** N35° 56.433' W105° 23.733'

# 10

# Sugarite Canyon State Park

*Rated as one of the most magnificent state parks in New Mexico*

**S**ugarite Canyon State Park's property borders the state of Colorado, and elevations range from 6,900 feet at the park entrance to 8,320 feet atop Little Horse Mesa. Sugarite Canyon came within a hairbreadth of being burned completely to the ground by the Track Wildfire. On June 12, 2011, the Track fire was listed as caused by humans and burned 27,792 acres before it was fully contained on June 29, 2011. You will see tree damage along the Soda Pocket Road, but thankfully, this beautiful campground was spared.

Within Sugarite Canyon's boundaries lie two beautiful lakes, Lake Alice and Lake Maloya. Lake Maloya's northern edge reaches into Colorado. There is no camping at Lake Maloya, but the Lake Alice Campground is slightly north of the lake on the west side of the road. Lake Alice is a small lake of 3 water acres, while Lake Maloya stretches out over 130 acres. Because Lake Maloya is the water supply for the city of Raton, there is no swimming, but sailboats, fishing boats with electric trolling motors,

canoes, kayaks, and rafts are allowed. Both lakes are well stocked with rainbow trout.

The park is home to an old coal camp, accessible from a trail beginning behind the visitor center. This hike is approximately 1.5 miles and considered moderate to strenuous. Nine other hiking trails are in the park; information and maps of all hiking trails are available at the visitor center. Across from the visitor center is the comfort station, with flush toilets and warm-water showers. The facilities are kept extremely clean.

Two campgrounds are within Sugarite Canyon State Park. Lake Alice Campground (across the road from the lake) is ideal for RVs, with water and electrical hookups. This camp is alongside the park road, so road noise is a factor. All sites are shady but tightly compacted. All new pit toilets have been installed at the Lake Alice Campground.

The turnoff for Soda Pocket Campground is 1 mile north of Lake Alice on the left. This well-maintained gravel road curves uphill, gaining 497 feet in elevation. Arriving at Soda Pocket you will find a family-friendly campground that is ideal for tent campers. All sites here are on a first-come, first-serve basis. The main camp begins along a long gravel road and ends in a large loop. Many sites are shady under a thickly forested canopy of Gambel oak, interspersed with ponderosa pine, juniper, and cedar trees. The majority of sites here are large and private, with most separated with scrub oak and

## :: Ratings

BEAUTY: ★ ★ ★ ★ ★
PRIVACY: ★ ★ ★ ★ ★
SPACIOUSNESS: ★ ★ ★ ★ ★
QUIET: ★ ★ ★ ★ ★
SECURITY: ★ ★ ★ ★ ★
CLEANLINESS: ★ ★ ★ ★ ★

## :: Key Information

**ADDRESS:** 211 Hwy. 526, Raton, NM 87740

**OPERATED BY:** New Mexico State Parks

**CONTACT:** 575-445-5607; **www.emnrd .state.nm.us/SPD/sugaritecanyonstate park.html**

**OPEN:** Year-round

**SITES:** 40, plus Gambel Oak group camp and Ponderosa Horse Camp

**SITE AMENITIES:** Parking space, picnic table, fire ring; some have pedestal grills, shade shelters, and bear-proof food-storage lockers.

**ASSIGNMENT:** Some Lake Alice sites and the group camp can be reserved at **reserveamerica.com** or 877-664-7787; all other sites are first come, first served.

**REGISTRATION:** Self-registration on-site without a reservation; with reservation, follow instructions on website and print receipt of reservation for check-in.

**FACILITIES:** Amphitheater, boat dock and ramp, restrooms with showers, vault toilets, visitor center

**PARKING:** At site

**FEE:** $10 nonelectric, $14 with electric or sewage hookup, $18 with electric and sewage hookups; $5 day-use fee per vehicle

**ELEVATION:** *Lake Alice* 7,142 feet; *Soda Pocket entrance road* 7,891 feet

**RESTRICTIONS**

■ **Pets:** On 10-foot leash; take precautionary measures against predators

■ **Fires:** In fire rings only; charcoal grills permitted; check with campground host, Forest Service office, and postings on camp bulletin board for restrictions.

■ **Alcohol:** At campsites only; glass not permitted

■ **Other:** Quiet hours 10 p.m.–8 a.m.; 14-day stay limit

other bushes. The sites that are not under the tree canopy are equipped with steel shelters over the picnic tables. Some sites are equipped with bear boxes—please use them—and several sites have pedestal grills. RVs are allowed to camp here, but generator use is not permitted during quiet hours. The two vault toilets in the camp are brand new. On my visit, the water system at Soda Pocket was not yet complete, so you might need to get water at Lake Alice Campground. There is no firewood to be gathered here, so it's best to bring your own or buy firewood in Raton.

The campground hosts keep the camp secure, locking the gate at sunset every evening and providing everyone with the gate combination numbers to get in and out of camp. Frequent patrols by park rangers add to the security here.

*Warning:* Bears are abundant in this area, and several individual bears are known to frequent the park. If your site has a bear box, use it. If not, pack all food items in your vehicle every night, and keep a clean camp. To ensure your safety, follow instructions in this book on page 10 and all instructions posted on the campground bulletin board. If you have questions about bears in this area, consult the park staff.

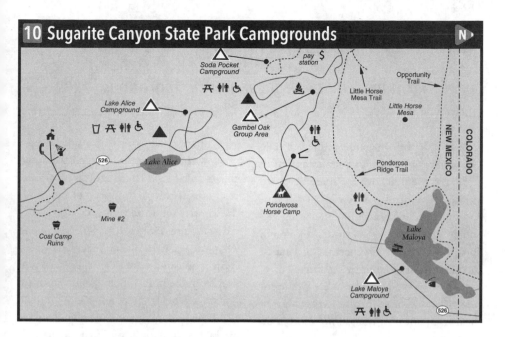

## 10 Sugarite Canyon State Park Campgrounds

## :: Getting There

From Raton, drive west on NM 72 for 3 miles, turn north on NM 526 and go 2 miles to park entrance. Lake Alice Campground entrance is 0.75 miles north of the park visitor center, and the Soda Pocket Campground road entrance is 1 mile farther north.

**GPS COORDINATES**   N36° 57.548'   W104° 23.189'

# 11

# Valle Vidal Campgrounds

*Peace, harmony, and two equestrian campgrounds*

**V**alle Vidal (meaning Valley of Life in Spanish) is a lush mountain basin located in the heart of the Sangre de Cristo Mountains of northern New Mexico. Abundant populations of wildlife, including elk, buffalo, mule deer, black bears, mountain lions, bald eagles, and native Rio Grande cutthroat trout, inhabit this protected area. Vast alpine meadows of the Valle Vidal provide critical habitat for the largest herd of elk in New Mexico, numbering more than 2,000 animals.

## CIMARRON CAMPGROUND

Beautiful Cimarron Campground is the more pristine of the two campgrounds in Valle Vidal. Surrounded by towering ponderosa pine, aspen, blue spruce, and Douglas fir trees, this lovely place is an equestrian camper's dream. There will be some RVs here, but the camp is quiet and majestic. A campground host is assigned here, and the New Mexico Department of Game and Fish patrols this area frequently, so security is excellent.

Cimarron is divided into two separate loops, with two vault toilets and two water spigots per loop. There are varmint-proof trash bins within and outside of the camp. The camp is set up with private, roomy sites and some grass. Sites 2, 3, 5–11, 13, 20, and 26–35 are designated as nonequestrian sites. Those who camp with dogs must keep pets away from the horses. Sites 3 and 17 are designated as wheelchair accessible.

Trails are open to equestrians, mountain bikers, and hikers, and there are literally dozens from which to choose, rated from easy to difficult. Nearby, Shuree Ponds are stocked with rainbow trout, and the adjoining Shuree and Ponil Creeks can be fished for Rio Grande cutthroat trout.

This camp is set at more than 9,500 feet in elevation, and the temperatures dip into the low 40°F range most nights. Days are mild, never exceeding the mid-80s. Frequent thunderstorms occur here, and lightning is common. Due to its remoteness, black bears frequent this camp, and mountain lions and bobcats can be present. Coyotes can be heard nearly every night.

## :: Ratings

| *Cimarron* |
| --- |
| BEAUTY: ★ ★ ★ ★ ★ |
| PRIVACY: ★ ★ ★ |
| SPACIOUSNESS: ★ ★ ★ ★ |
| QUIET: ★ ★ ★ ★ |
| SECURITY: ★ ★ ★ ★ |
| CLEANLINESS: ★ ★ ★ ★ |

| *McCrystal* |
| --- |
| BEAUTY: ★ ★ ★ ★ |
| PRIVACY: ★ ★ ★ ★ |
| SPACIOUSNESS: ★ ★ ★ ★ |
| QUIET: ★ ★ ★ ★ |
| SECURITY: ★ ★ ★ |
| CLEANLINESS: ★ ★ ★ |

## :: Key Information

**ADDRESS:** Carson National Forest, Questa Ranger District, P.O. Box 10, Questa, NM 87556

**OPERATED BY:** U.S. Department of Agriculture

**CONTACT:** 575-586-0520; **www.fs.usda.gov/carson**

**OPEN:** May–Oct., weather permitting

**SITES:** *Cimarron* 35; *McCrystal* 60

**SITE AMENITIES:** Parking space, picnic table, fire ring; equestrian sites equipped with corrals and grain bins

**ASSIGNMENT:** *Cimarron:* first come, first served or reserve at **reserveamerica.com** or **recreation.gov**; *McCrystal:* first come, first served only

**REGISTRATION:** Self-registration on-site without a reservation; with reservation, follow instructions on website and print receipt of reservation for check-in.

**FACILITIES:** Vault toilets

**PARKING:** At site

**FEE:** *Cimarron* $16 single, $30 double; *McCrystal* $12; $5 per extra vehicle

**ELEVATION:** *Cimarron* 9,400 feet; *McCrystal* 8,144 feet

**RESTRICTIONS**

■ **Pets:** On 6-foot leash; take precautionary measures against predators; keep pets away from horses

■ **Fires:** In fire rings; charcoal grills permitted; check with campground host, Forest Service office, and postings on the camp bulletin board for restrictions.

■ **Alcohol:** At campsites only

■ **Other:** Quiet hours 10 p.m.–8 a.m.; 14-day stay limit

## MCCRYSTAL CAMPGROUND

McCrystal Campground is a lovely place for those who want to enjoy peace and harmony and horses. Set in a tall forest of ponderosa pines with abundant wildflowers, it's located off Forest Service Road 1950.

This camp is very large, and all sites are level. Most sites are grassy, shady, and well spaced with plenty of room. Equestrian sites are larger, with corrals and grain bins, and are marked. This campground boasts 60 campsites equally spaced apart in three large loops. McCrystal is used frequently by the Boy Scouts from nearby Philmont Scout Ranch. It is best to call the Questa Ranger Station before planning a trip, as more than 2,000 Scouts use this camp throughout the summer.

There is no potable water here, so you must bring in your own. Several stock tanks supply horses with water, but it is not potable for human use. There is plenty of firewood to gather outside of the campground along the roadway. Security is good, and although there is no host here, the Forest Service patrols this area along with leaders from the Philmont Scout Ranch. Due to the remoteness of this campground, there is very little traffic, so you won't experience much road noise. All campsites are set back far enough away from the road that dust clouds are not a factor. Due to the level sites, almost all sites are wheelchair accessible; however, the four portable toilets that service the campground are not.

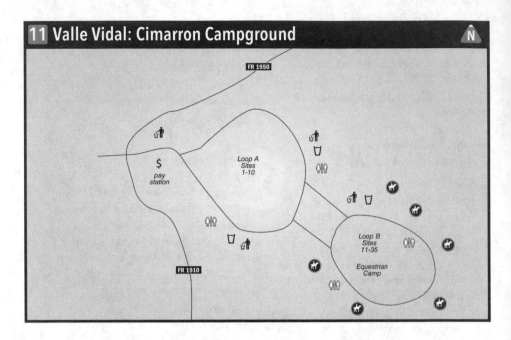

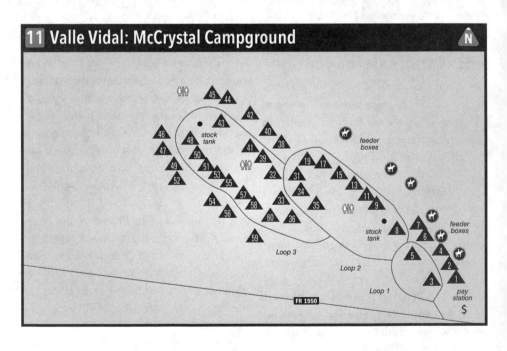

# :: Getting There

## CIMARRON

July 1 through end of November: From Costilla, travel east on NM 196 past Amalia, to the intersection of FR 1950. Travel 10 miles on FR 1950 (a gravel road) east to the junction with FR 1910. Cimarron Campground is 1 mile uphill to the right. (This gate is closed during elk calving season, from April 1 through June 30.)

April 1 through June 30: From NM 64, 9 miles east of Cimarron, NM, turn north on FR 1950 for 35 miles to FR 1910. (This gate is closed January 1 through March 1 to prevent stress on wintering elk herds.)

## McCRYSTAL

July 1 through end of November: From Costilla, travel east on NM 196 past Amalia, to the intersection of FR 1950. Travel approximately 30 miles on FR 1950 to the campground. (This gate is closed during elk calving season, from April 1 through June 30.)

April 1 through June 30: From NM 64, 9 miles east of Cimarron, NM, turn north on FR 1950 for 35 miles to the campground entrance on the right. (This gate is closed January 1 through March 1 to prevent stress on wintering elk herds.)

Note: These gravel roads are not maintained during the rainy season and may be passable only with a four-wheel-drive vehicle.

### GPS COORDINATES

**Cimarron**   N36° 46.203'   W105° 12.347'

**McCrystal**   N36° 46.607'   W105° 6.942'

# 12

# Rio Grande del Norte National Monument

*Check out these two brand-new campground complexes within the new Rio Grande del Norte National Monument.*

**T**he Rio Grande was among the original eight rivers selected in 1968 by Congress as Wild and Scenic. The designated river area includes 56 miles of the Rio Grande, from the New Mexico state line to beyond the Orilla Verde Recreation Site. The Rio Grande begins in the snowcapped Rocky Mountains of Colorado, journeys south through New Mexico, and farther south carves the border between Texas and Mexico. From its beginnings in Colorado, it travels 1,900 miles to the Gulf of Mexico. The Upper Rio Grande passes through the 800-foot-deep Rio Grande Gorge, creating a rugged and majestic playground for those who love the wild outdoors.

The canyon is filled with exciting recreational opportunities, luring fishermen and whitewater rafting and boating enthusiasts. The magnificent Rio Grande Gorge area attracts photographers and artists, many local, and others from as far away as you can imagine.

Hikers can choose from 36 miles of marked trails; most are easy to moderate, except the Picuris Trail, which is only 0.8 mile but rated difficult. Most trails accommodate mountain bikes and horses, as well as hikers. The canyon trails are lined with lava rock, which is sharp and jagged; this is not a good place to fall. Stay hydrated during hikes and know your limits.

Be careful if you venture onto the river; the currents are strong, dangerous, and cold, and will challenge any whitewater expert. Two popular whitewater sections are the Taos Box, which consists of 17 miles of Class IV whitewater, run from late April to mid-July; and the 5-mile Racecourse, a Class III segment that is great running from May through August.

Please become familiar with the river's dangers by stopping at the visitor centers for very important safety information. Because of rapidly changing weather and potential flash flooding, the Rio Grande's demeanor can change very quickly. Check weather

## :: Ratings

### Orilla Verde Campgrounds
BEAUTY: ★ ★ ★ ★
PRIVACY: ★ ★ ★ ★
SPACIOUSNESS: ★ ★ ★
QUIET: ★ ★ ★ ★
SECURITY: ★ ★ ★ ★ ★
CLEANLINESS: ★ ★ ★ ★ ★

### Wild Rivers Campgrounds
BEAUTY: ★ ★ ★ ★
PRIVACY: ★ ★ ★ ★
SPACIOUSNESS: ★ ★ ★ ★
QUIET: ★ ★ ★ ★ ★
SECURITY: ★ ★ ★ ★ ★
CLEANLINESS: ★ ★ ★ ★ ★

## :: Key Information

**ADDRESS:** BLM Taos Field Office, 226 Cruz Alta Rd., Taos, NM 87571-5983

**OPERATED BY:** Bureau of Land Management

**CONTACT:** 575-758-8851; **blm.gov**

**OPEN:** Year-round, but snow can temporarily restrict access in winter.

**SITES:** *Orilla Verde* 7 campgrounds with 48 sites; *Wild Rivers* 5 campgrounds with 26 sites

**SITE AMENITIES:** Parking space, picnic table, fire ring

**ASSIGNMENT:** First come, first served

**REGISTRATION:** Self-registration on-site

**FACILITIES:** Visitor centers

**PARKING:** At each site

**FEE:** $7/night for 1 vehicle, $10/night for 2; maximum 2 vehicles and 8 people allowed per site; additional vehicles may park in day-use parking areas at $3/day; $15/night for water and electrical hookups; $5/night for primitive sites

**ELEVATION:** *Orilla Verde* 6,459 feet; *Wild Rivers* 7,571 feet

**RESTRICTIONS**

■ **Pets:** On 6-ft. leash; this is black bear country and also home to mountain lions, bobcats, and coyotes, so monitor pets closely.

■ **Fires:** In fire rings only; charcoal grills permitted; check with campground host, BLM office, and postings on the camp bulletin board for restrictions; firewood is available from campground hosts, at the visitor center, and in Pilar, Taos, or Questa.

■ **Alcohol:** At campsites only

■ **Other:** Quiet hours 10 p.m.–8 a.m.; 14-day stay limit

---

forecasts frequently, and know your limits, skill level, and equipment limitations.

### ORILLA VERDE CAMPGROUNDS

The Orilla Verde Recreation Area is a great place for you to select from any one of seven campgrounds situated along the upper Rio Grande Wild and Scenic River. The newly remodeled campgrounds are mostly shady, thanks to the tree-lined riverbanks, and many of the sites that lack trees have sun shelters. All campgrounds have numbered sites with tables, fire rings, and restrooms. And all have water except Rio Puebla Primitive Campground.

Remember this is New Mexico, so bring high-SPF sunscreen, stay hydrated, and expect temperatures in the 90s during the day. The canyon sees the sun's rays later in the morning, and loses the sunlight earlier in the afternoon. The steep canyon walls provide cool early mornings and comfortable nights.

From the Rio Grande Gorge Visitor Center, you will encounter the campgrounds in the following order:

**PILAR CAMPGROUND:** 14 sites (9 RV sites with water and electric, 5 tent sites), 6 shelters; 1 restroom with flushable toilet, 1 vault toilet; no tree shade across the road from the river.

**RIO BRAVO CAMPGROUND:** 11 sites (4 RV sites with water and electric, 7 tent sites), 1 group shelter; 1 restroom with flush toilets, coin pay shower, 1 vault toilet; 7 shelters and excellent tree shade on all riverside-facing sites.

**ARROYO HONDO CAMPGROUND:** 4 RV/tent sites; no water, electricity, or shelters and very little tree shade; riverside camping; 1 vault toilet.

**LONE JUNIPER CAMPGROUND:** 4 RV/tent sites; no water, electricity, or shelters and little tree shade; riverside camping; 1 vault toilet; boat ramp.

**PETACA CAMPGROUND:** 5 sites, 3 shelters; water available; 1 vault toilet; good cluster of trees for shade; across the road from the river.

**TAOS JUNCTION CAMPGROUND:** 4 sites with water, large group shelter with electricity and water; riverside camping; 1 restroom with water and 1 vault toilet.

**RIO PUEBLA PRIMITIVE CAMPGROUND:** 6 sites with picnic tables and fire rings; 1 vault toilet; no water; Rio Puebla offers little to no shade, so a portable sun canopy is highly recommended.

## WILD RIVERS CAMPGROUNDS

The Wild Rivers Recreation Area campgrounds offer a totally different environment than the Orilla Verde campgrounds. You could say the Wild Rivers campgrounds give you "a room with a view." Instead of camping at the bottom of the canyon as at the Orilla Verde camps, you will be camping 800 feet high on the rim of a very steep, very wide crevice in the earth. If you are a sleepwalker, you might want to opt for another camping area.

When you look down into the canyon, the vertical walls are covered with cedar, piñon, and juniper trees and yucca plants, silver sage, and cacti. The hearty plants that grow in this deep terrain are drought tolerant and cast a colorful hue on the canyon walls that are composed of black lava rock. When you look off to the southeast, you will see the beautiful mountains that encompass the Taos Ski Area and the mountains that form the Red River valley to the east.

Numerous campsites at the bottom of the canyon can only be reached by backpacking. These canyon-bottom sites are accessed via trailheads that start at the different campgrounds. These sites are obviously pack in/pack out camping. You will see numerous switchback trails that backpackers use to access these remote sites.

The new Wild Rivers Visitor Center provides great information about the area, including maps for hikers. The staff members at all of the visitor centers are very helpful and friendly. There are more than 30 miles of marked trails from the campgrounds. Two trails are considered easy, seven are listed as moderate, and two are considered difficult. Please keep well hydrated while on the trail, watch your step, and do not exceed your hiking capabilities. Sunscreen and a hat are essential on the trail, and all trails will test your endurance. Be on constant watch for rattlesnakes in the campgrounds and trail areas.

*Note:* There are no RV hookups at any of the campgrounds in the Wild Rivers Recreation Area.

From the Wild Rivers Visitor Center, you will encounter the campgrounds in the following order:

**EL AGUAJE CAMPGROUND:** 7 sites with shelters, 1 host site, group shelter accommodates 30; 1 vault toilet.

**LA JUNTA POINT CAMPGROUND:** 3 sites within the loop with shelters, plus several primitive sites along the La Junta Overlook Trail, which are set up without shelters, but are equipped with tables and fire rings. The oval-shaped trail takes you around the primitive sites to a spectacular overlook over

## 12 Rio Grande del Norte N.M.: Orilla Verde Campgrounds

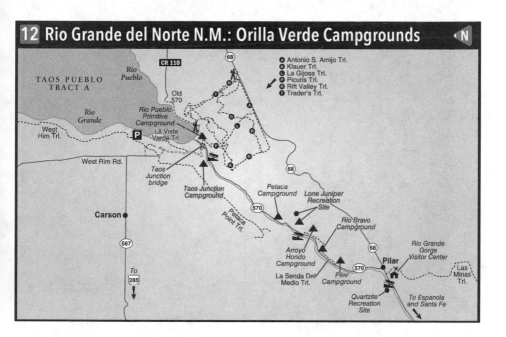

the Rio Grande Gorge. You are right at the edge of an 800-foot cliff, and the views are breathtaking. The trail to the overlook is wheelchair accessible. This campground sits on the pointed edge of the arrowhead-shaped cliff to the east, and the Red River Gorge to the west. This is the place at the bottom of the canyon where the Red River flows into the Rio Grande. If you view the campground on Google Earth, you will see the arrowhead-shaped point. The campground is equipped with vault toilets.

**MONTOSO CAMPGROUND:** 4 sites with shelters; no water; vault toilets; overlooks the Rio Grande Gorge.

**LITTLE ARSENIC CAMPGROUND:** 6 sites with shelters; water and vault toilets.

**BIG ARSENIC SPRINGS CAMPGROUND:** 5 sites with shelters; vault toilets, water, fire pits; 1 shelter is for day use by parking area and the trailhead.

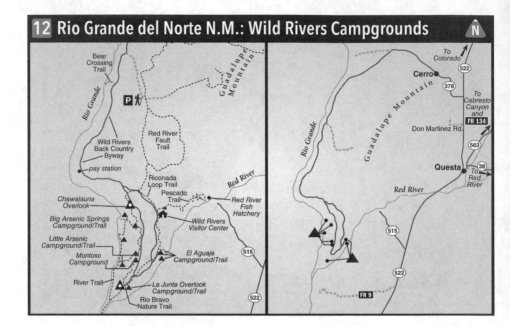

## 12 Rio Grande del Norte N.M.: Wild Rivers Campgrounds

## :: Getting There

### ORILLA VERDE

From Taos, travel 16.5 miles southwest on NM 68 to Pilar, NM. Turn right on NM 570 and follow it to each of the campgrounds. The campgrounds are listed from south to north, which is the most common way to enter the Orilla Verde Recreation Area. The visitor center is just a short 0.25 mile south of the NM 570 junction.

### WILD RIVERS

From Taos, follow NM 68 north 7 miles. Take NM 522 approximately 20 miles to Questa. Travel 3 miles past the stoplight in Questa to NM 378. Turn left onto NM 378 and follow the signs about 12 miles west to Wild Rivers Recreation Area.

#### GPS COORDINATES

**Rio Grande Gorge Visitor Center**   N36° 16.064'   W105° 47.383'

**Wild Rivers Visitor Center**   N36° 40.878'   W105° 40.384'

# 13

# San Antonio Campground

*Families love this campground with open areas where children can play.*

**San Antonio** Campground is a tent-camper's delight. Named for San Antonio Creek, which flows through camp, this mountain oasis fills to the brim every weekend between Memorial Day and Labor Day; reservations are highly recommended. The campground was completely rebuilt and reopened in August 2010. A paved walking trail along the river provides stream access for fishing. Anglers have landed some impressive rainbow trout here.

This campground is designated as a reduced-impact and recycle campground. Users are encouraged to recycle (recycle bins on-site) and pack out trash. Cutting live vegetation is prohibited.

A campground host is assigned to San Antonio, and Forest Service officers and the Sandoval County Sheriff's Department frequently patrol this campground, so you will be safe here. New Mexico Department of Game and Fish wardens frequently check for fishing licenses and catch limits at this campground.

San Antonio has two separate tent areas, set away from the RV sites. Sites 11–19 are located on the north end of the campground and are tent-only, walk-in sites. Several sites on the north end are wheelchair accessible, and the vault toilet at the north end of the campground is equipped with a wheelchair ramp. There is also a wheelchair-accessible fishing spot by the stream. Four pit toilets are located within an easy walk of all campsites. Three additional walk-in sites and a large open meadow are located on the south end of the campground. Site GA and site 26 (no electric hookups on either site) are designated for disabled campers.

Tent campers are allowed to use individual sites along the road, but you may end up camping next to an RV. Sites 1–6 are equipped with 50-amp electrical hookups. Because this is a small campground, privacy is nearly nonexistent. The campground is right along NM 126, so traffic noise can be an irritant. And on weekends, San Antonio gets really crowded with traffic; watch your children and pets carefully. Despite these drawbacks, the campground is quite shady with large mature ponderosa pines.

Families love it here, and there are open areas where children can play. The stream is pleasant to fish or soak your feet in. Crossing the stream, you will find several hiking trails winding up the side of the mountain.

If you love hummingbirds, bring your feeder. The New Mexico mountains are

## :: Ratings

BEAUTY: ★ ★ ★ ★
PRIVACY: ★
SPACIOUSNESS: ★ ★
QUIET: ★
SECURITY: ★ ★ ★ ★ ★
CLEANLINESS: ★ ★ ★

## :: Key Information

**ADDRESS:** Santa Fe National Forest, Jemez Ranger District, P.O. Box 150, Jemez Springs, NM 87025

**OPERATED BY:** U.S. Department of Agriculture

**CONTACT:** 575-829-3535; www.fs.usda.gov/santafe

**OPEN:** Before Memorial Day–after Labor Day, depending on weather

**SITES:** 30, 6 with electric and water hookups

**SITE AMENITIES:** Parking space, picnic table, fire ring

**ASSIGNMENT:** Sites 1–10, 20–26, and GA (disabled site) can be reserved at reserveamerica.com or recreation.gov; sites 11–19 are first come, first served only.

**REGISTRATION:** Self-registration on-site without a reservation; with reservation, follow instructions on website and print receipt of reservation for check-in.

**FACILITIES:** Vault toilets

**PARKING:** At each site

**FEE:** $10, $15 with electrical hookup

**ELEVATION:** 8,171 feet

**RESTRICTIONS**

■ **Pets:** On 6-foot leash; take precautionary measures against predators; bear tracks are spotted occasionally along the San Antonio River.

■ **Fires:** In fire rings only; charcoal grills permitted, but no firewood in pedestal cooking grills

■ **Alcohol:** At campsites only

■ **Other:** Quiet hours 10 p.m.–8 a.m.; 14-day stay limit

home to broad-tailed hummingbirds. You will occasionally spot rufous hummingbirds, which are territorial and may chase off the broad-tailed ones. American crows are residents in the forest here, too. Blue jays frequent the campground, as do Steller's jays. Chipmunks scurry about the campground and are fun to feed.

This is one of few areas in which mosquitoes are a problem in the Jemez Mountains, so bring insect repellent. Nightly raids by raccoons are also irritating. These masked bandits are not shy at all and are adept at stealing food. Keep all food items in your vehicle. Bears are spotted at this campground every year. I have seen bear tracks by the stream numerous times. Take the necessary precautions, and read and obey the alerts posted at the camp.

The community of La Cueva has a nice little store called Amanda's; it's well stocked with whatever you might have forgotten to pack from home, including ice, dry firewood, fishing tackle, and New Mexico fishing licenses. The owner, Ray, keeps the prices reasonable. Cellular service here can be spotty, but Amanda's will allow you to make calls from a phone by the cash register for a modest fee. Next door, The Ridgeback Cafe serves great food if you tire of camp cooking.

Hot springs are popular in the Jemez Wilderness. McCauley Warm Springs is a 1.5-mile hike from nearby Battleship Rock picnic grounds. San Antonio Hot Springs is by far the best. From the campground, drive north 3 miles on NM 126, and then turn right onto Forest Service Road 376 for 6 bumpy miles; the road ends at the parking lot. Walk across

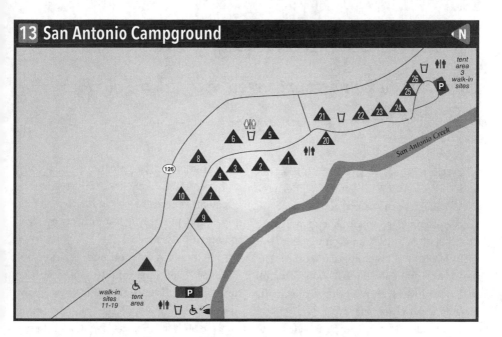

## 13 San Antonio Campground

a railroad-tie bridge and hike up a fairly steep incline 100 yards to the pools. Many families visit these hot springs, and the crowds are well behaved. A few miles south of the campground is a paved parking lot for Spence Hot Springs, but this spring is a disappointment. Litter, broken beer bottles, and beer cans are strewn along the rugged uphill trail and all around the hot spring pools. Nudity is the rule rather than the exception, and drugs and alcohol are frequently consumed in the open at this location.

## :: Getting There

From the ranger station in Jemez Springs, drive north on US 4. Turn left (north) at the La Cueva Junction onto NM 126. After 2 miles, turn left (east) into the campground.

**GPS COORDINATES**   N35° 53.168'   W106° 38.783'

# 14

# Redondo Campground

*This beautiful campground greets you with the glorious fragrance of pine.*

**R**edondo **Campground** boasts all the beauty of the Jemez Wilderness. Encapsulated within a mature forest of tall ponderosa pines, scattered aspens, and other mixed conifers, this campground greets you with the glorious fragrance of the pines. The meadows within Redondo's boundaries fill with wildflowers every spring, continually blooming until frost sets in.

Redondo Campground is close to my heart because it is the first place that I camped after moving to New Mexico in August of 1988. It is also the first place my wife Susan, stepson Chris, and I camped after our wedding in 1990. Every year I make my pilgrimage back to this lovely environment.

Redondo Campground is named for the 11,254-foot Redondo Peak, visible to the east. Redondo boasts the highest elevation among the Jemez campgrounds at 8,180 feet above sea level, so prepare for summer nights in the 40°F–50°F range. Afternoon showers occur frequently during the New Mexico monsoon season, which begins in July and continues through September. Violent lightning storms

are common, so be prepared to take cover. Summer days rarely exceed the mid-80s. Frequent breezes bend the huge ponderosa pines and perform a beautiful forest symphony through the forest.

Redondo is wonderful for children and families. The campground road is exactly 1 mile in length, encompassing three loops. It's perfect for a bicycle ride, skateboarding, or a leisurely stroll. Kids love it, and there is plenty of space for them to play.

The Redondo well went dry in 2003, but water is available at nearby San Antonio Campground. Future plans are to drill a new well and remodel the campground whenever the federal budget allocates the funds to the Forest Service. Recent forest thinning for fire protection at this campground has not detracted from the beauty of the area, and there is a significant amount of firewood available.

A campground host is assigned here from Memorial Day through Labor Day. Forest Service officers and the Sandoval County Sheriff's Department patrol frequently, so you will be secure at Redondo Campground.

Privacy and spaciousness at this campground will vary. Most of the campsites on the inside of the loops are too closely spaced, whereas the sites on the outside will provide more solitude. RV campers frequent this campground, but there are many places to pitch your tent away from other campers and enjoy your privacy. Most sites

## :: Ratings

BEAUTY: ★ ★ ★ ★ ★
PRIVACY: ★ ★ ★
SPACIOUSNESS: ★ ★ ★ ★
QUIET: ★ ★
SECURITY: ★ ★ ★ ★ ★
CLEANLINESS: ★ ★ ★

## :: Key Information

**ADDRESS:** Santa Fe National Forest, Jemez Ranger District, P.O. Box 150, Jemez Springs, NM 87025

**OPERATED BY:** U.S. Department of Agriculture

**CONTACT:** 575-829-3535; www.fs.usda.gov/santafe

**OPEN:** Mid-May–mid-Sept.

**SITES:** 60

**SITE AMENITIES:** Parking space, picnic table, fire ring

**ASSIGNMENT:** First come, first served

**REGISTRATION:** Self-registration on-site

**FACILITIES:** Vault toilet

**PARKING:** At each site

**FEE:** $10

**ELEVATION:** 8,180 feet

**RESTRICTIONS**

■ **Pets:** On 6-foot leash; take precautionary measures against predators

■ **Fires:** In fire rings only; charcoal grills permitted; check with campground host, Forest Service office, and postings on the camp bulletin board for restrictions.

■ **Alcohol:** At campsites only

■ **Other:** Quiet hours 10 p.m.–8 a.m.

are shaded. Five vault toilets are distributed conveniently throughout the campground. A fair warning: these facilities are old and become quite putrid as the weather warms.

Flies, bees, and wasps are common here, but there are few mosquitoes or other bloodthirsty pests. You may see many varieties of butterflies, and various species of woodboring beetles frequently come for a visit.

If you love hummingbirds, bring your feeder. The New Mexico mountains are home to broad-tailed hummingbirds. You will occasionally spot rufous hummingbirds, which are territorial and may chase off the broad-tailed birds. American crows are residents in the forest here, too, as are blue jays and Steller's jays.

Mule deer, elk, coyotes, black bears, mountain lions, and bobcats all make their homes in the surrounding mountain areas. In spring, deer and elk droppings are commonly found within the campground, but they migrate to higher elevations as summer approaches. Be careful driving down NM 4—wildlife cross this road frequently. There have been no reported sightings of predatory animals within the campgrounds, but be wary because this is black bear country.

There are two hiking and mountain biking trails inside this campground. The Redondo Loop is a 2.5-mile round-trip, and the Redondo Campground Trail is a 2-mile hike. Both are considered easy to moderate.

Off-road motorcycles and ATVs are permitted in a limited area of the Jemez Wilderness. Stop by the Jemez Ranger Station to obtain detailed information regarding motorized vehicles before proceeding and be aware that rules may change frequently. Drive your off-road vehicle carefully; hikers, mountain bikers, and equestrians travel in areas where off-road vehicles are permitted.

Redondo Campground has an amphitheater, and it gets a significant amount of use. In the past, college students interning with the Forest Service have given nature talks on a wide variety of subjects. I have attended programs on wildlife spotting, big cats of the Southwest, owls, native cutthroat trout, and wildfire prevention. It is a really worthwhile educational program—ideal for kids—and the interns make it fun.

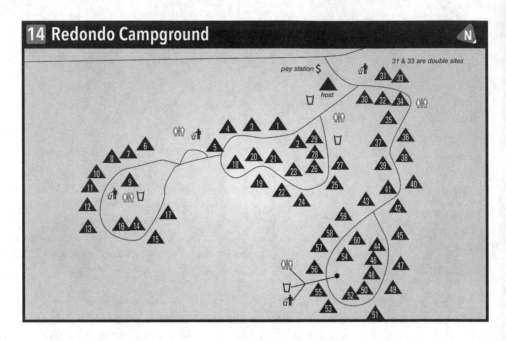

## :: Getting There

From Jemez Ranger Station, drive north on US 4 for 9.5 miles, and turn left into the campground.

**GPS COORDINATES**  N35° 51.653'  W106° 37.680'

# 15

# Jemez Falls Campground

*This jewel of a campground is the pride of the Jemez area.*

**L**ocated in a valley surrounded by towering ponderosa pines and aspens, Jemez Falls Campground is the pride of the Jemez area. It's one of the newer campgrounds in the Jemez Wilderness and is sparkling clean. Tents and RVs cohabitate well at this campground, and pop-up campers and trailers are common. With many large campsites and generous spacing between sites, your time spent here will be peaceful. Of all the campgrounds in this book, this is my number one choice.

Four loops exist within the campground, and the large RVs tend to prefer the loop to the far right. This loop is the closest to NM 4 and receives some highway noise. Due to the campground topography and distance from the highway, highway noise is not a factor on the other loops.

Tent campers have many delightful spaces, and most spots are grassy, level, and shaded by the dense canopy of ponderosa pines. You will notice outcroppings of young ponderosas throughout the campground. Forest thinning took place here several years ago but did not detract from the forest's beauty.

## :: Ratings

BEAUTY: ★ ★ ★ ★ ★
PRIVACY: ★ ★ ★ ★
SPACIOUSNESS: ★ ★ ★ ★ ★
QUIET: ★ ★ ★ ★
SECURITY: ★ ★ ★ ★ ★
CLEANLINESS: ★ ★ ★ ★ ★

Four new vault toilets are distributed conveniently and kept spotless. Jemez Falls has an underground pressurized well, and the water from the well is treated. Water spigots are located near each toilet.

This campground is popular, so get here as early as possible if you're visiting on a weekend. Even when the campground is full, it's surprisingly quiet. Camping here during the week is phenomenal if you love serenity.

You will see plenty of blue jays, several species of woodpeckers, and a large population of hummingbirds.

This is bear country, so read and adhere to the posted signs. Bobcats, mountain lions, and coyotes are also common carnivores here. If you bring pets, keep them on a leash at all times and be wary. Deer and elk herds frequent this area but migrate to remote areas in the Santa Fe National Forest when camping season arrives. Be careful driving down NM 4 because wildlife cross this road frequently.

Jemez Falls has an amphitheater, and there is a nondenominational church service held every Sunday morning at 8 a.m. In the past, Forest Service interns have also put on educational nature programs at the amphitheater.

Kids love this campground, and there are plenty of places where they can play safely. The 1.5-mile road through the campground has a few hills and is an easy, fun bicycle ride. The speed limit is posted at 10 miles per hour and strictly enforced.

## :: Key Information

**ADDRESS:** Santa Fe National Forest, Jemez Ranger District, P.O. Box 150, Jemez Springs, NM 87025

**OPERATED BY:** U.S. Department of Agriculture

**CONTACT:** 575-829-3535; www.fs.usda.gov/santafe

**OPEN:** May–mid-Sept.

**SITES:** 52

**SITE AMENITIES:** Parking space, picnic table, fire ring

**ASSIGNMENT:** First come, first served

**REGISTRATION:** Self-registration on-site

**FACILITIES:** Vault toilets, amphitheater; bring water

**PARKING:** At each site

**FEE:** $10 single, $20 double

**ELEVATION:** 8,007 feet

**RESTRICTIONS**

■ **Pets:** On 6-foot leash

■ **Fires:** In fire rings only; charcoal grills permitted

■ **Alcohol:** At campsites only

■ **Other:** Quiet hours 10 p.m.–8 a.m.; 14-day stay limit

A campground host is on duty Memorial Day through Labor Day, and Forest Service officers and the Sandoval County Sheriff's Department patrol this campground often, so security is excellent here.

Jemez Falls may open as early as the first weekend in May, but the water is never turned on until the host arrives. The campground remains open until the end of September, but the Forest Service closes one or two of the loops as the crowds dwindle.

June 6, 2007, was a day that almost marked an end to this campground. After more than a week without rain, a terrible fire raged out of control and stopped within 50 feet of the campsites. The fire was apparently caused by heat lightning and jumped two fire lines before it was brought under control. The following Saturday afternoon, the rains came and soaked the lovely forest.

Outside the campground to the south, the Jemez Falls Trail leads to the majestic waterfalls. The 1-mile trail is easy to moderate, but the final descent to the falls is quite steep, so please exercise caution. At the end of the trail, a primitive log ladder provides access to the pool below the falls.

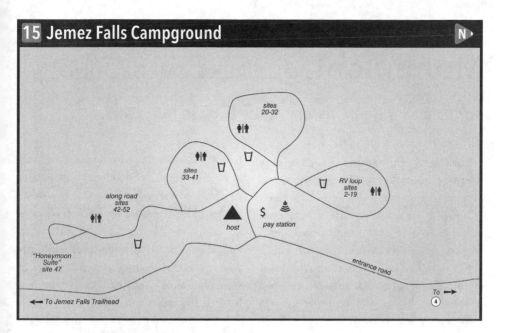

## :: Getting There

From Jemez Springs Ranger Station, drive north on NM 4 for 11.5 miles. Turn right at the Jemez Falls Campground sign and follow the road 1 mile to campground.

**GPS COORDINATES**   N35° 49.422'   W106° 36.368'

# 16

# Bandelier National Monument: JUNIPER CAMPGROUND

*Bandelier's human history dates back 10,000 years.*

**Juniper Campground** is an awesome place for a getaway. The campground is atop a volcanic mesa, dotted with juniper, piñon, and ponderosa pine trees. I gathered piñon nuts, a delightful camp snack. Juniper's 94 campsites are compressed within three loops, but some spots will afford you privacy. Some sites lack shade. I camped here in April on the east loop at site 8. It was ideal, with a large ponderosa pine for shade and a water spigot and restroom nearby. The restrooms are modern, with sinks and flush toilets, and kept spotless. The water is treated. Numerous sites are wheelchair accessible.

Gathering firewood is prohibited, but the camp host sells bundles of firewood, and plenty of firewood is available outside of the park along NM 4. National Park Service officers frequently patrol this campground, so you should be safe. Rules and policies are strictly adhered to, but the officers are friendly and helpful.

This is bear country, so abide by posted precautions. You may spot mountain lions, bobcats, coyotes, foxes, mule deer, wild turkeys, jackrabbits, chipmunks, and Abert's squirrels. In warm weather you may also see rattlesnakes. There are several species here, including the Western prairie rattlesnake and the Western diamondback. Educate yourself about venomous reptiles, watch your children closely, and keep your pets leashed and under control.

Summers here can be hot, reaching the upper 90s. Spring and fall are ideal seasons to visit, and the campground rarely fills up before Memorial Day or after Labor Day. Summer thunderstorms can be sudden and violent, so be ready to take cover. Spring weather is unpredictable, with cold nights until mid-May. Daytime temperatures in spring and fall are generally in the 50°F–60°F range. Fall camping is pleasant here through mid-October. Because this campground sits atop a mesa, it can get quite windy.

More than 70 miles of hiking trails wind throughout the national monument. The most popular hike begins at the visitor center and leads to Frijoles Canyon. You will find several excavation sites and the "cavates," a network of human-carved caves in the cliffside. The main archaeological sites were inhabited from the 1100s into the mid-1500s.

Those who love history and culture will appreciate that Bandelier's human history dates back 10,000 years, when nomadic hunters followed game through the canyons.

## :: Ratings

BEAUTY: ★ ★ ★ ★
PRIVACY: ★ ★ ★
SPACIOUSNESS: ★ ★ ★
QUIET: ★ ★ ★ ★ ★
SECURITY: ★ ★ ★ ★ ★
CLEANLINESS: ★ ★ ★ ★ ★

## :: Key Information

**ADDRESS:** Bandelier National Monument, 15 Entrance Rd., Los Alamos, NM 87544

**OPERATED BY:** National Park Service

**CONTACT:** 505-672-3861; nps.gov/band

**OPEN:** March 1–Oct. 31, weather permitting

**SITES:** 94

**SITE AMENITIES:** Parking space, picnic table, fire ring

**ASSIGNMENT:** First come, first served; only the 2 group sites may be reserved.

**REGISTRATION:** At electronic kiosk located at the entrance of the loops; select your site and then pay immediately; kiosk accepts credit cards or cash.

**FACILITIES:** Visitor center, restrooms, dump station

**PARKING:** At each site

**FEE:** $12; 7-day vehicle permit $12; Bandelier National Monument Annual Pass $30

**ELEVATION:** 6,672 feet at entrance

**RESTRICTIONS**

■ **Pets:** On 6-foot leash; not allowed on any trails within the park but permitted in the campground, picnic areas, and parking areas

■ **Fires:** In fire rings only; charcoal grills permitted; check with campground host, park office, and postings on the camp bulletin board for restrictions.

■ **Alcohol:** At campsites only

■ **Other:** Quiet hours 10 p.m.–6 a.m.; 14-day stay limit; limit of 2 tents, 2 vehicles, and 10 people per site

Ancestors of modern Pueblo people built thriving communities here 600 years ago. Remnants of several thousand dwellings have been found among the mesas and steep canyons. At the visitor center there is a snack bar, a gift shop, and a well-stocked bookstore. Interpretive ranger-led hikes are popular, as is the Bandelier Museum exhibit.

## 16 Bandelier National Monument: Juniper Campground

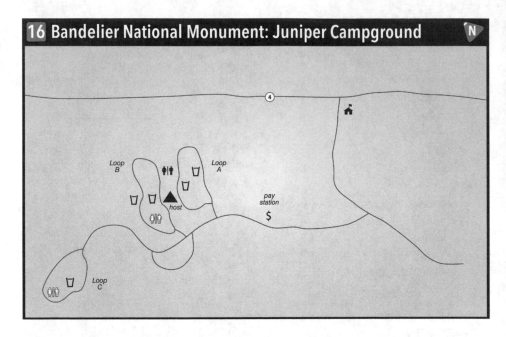

## :: Getting There

From Los Alamos, travel west on NM 4 for 11.5 miles, through the town of White Rock. Past White Rock, look for the large sign at the entrance to Bandelier National Monument.

**GPS COORDINATES**   N35° 47.712'   W106° 16.538'

# 17

# Fenton Lake State Park

*Many campers love to call this place home for the weekend.*

**F**enton Lake State Park was one of the most beautiful state parks in New Mexico until the Lakes Fire of August 27, 2002. This fire was started by a camper, and it destroyed more than 4,000 acres, including the ridge to the south, known as Lake Fork Mesa. The fire damage can be viewed from anywhere in the park. Fortunately, the campground was spared from the flames and is still a delightful place. Set in a deep forest of ponderosa pines, the campground remains beautiful, despite the surrounding areas devastated by the fire. Birdwatchers may spot Steller's jays, various woodpeckers, many hummingbirds, and raptors, including the peregrine falcon.

There is a large population of chipmunks, which love campers and can almost be fed by hand. Fenton Lake is also home to several species of ducks and geese, turkeys, mule deer, muskrats, elk, bobcats, mountain lions, coyotes, foxes, and black bears.

This state park does a good job separating RVs from tent campers. Loops A, B, and C are day-use areas. Loop D is the large RV loop. A sign beyond Loop D prohibits RVs from entering the tent-camper's loops.

## :: Ratings

BEAUTY: ★ ★ ★ ★ ★
PRIVACY: ★ ★ ★
SPACIOUSNESS: ★ ★ ★
QUIET: ★ ★ ★ ★
SECURITY: ★ ★ ★ ★ ★
CLEANLINESS: ★ ★ ★ ★ ★

Loops E and F are the areas tent campers call home. *Note:* the sites along the road are vulnerable to a cloud of fine dust every time a vehicle passes. The best sites are at the far end of the camp, away from traffic. The dusty road is the main drawback of camping at this park; asphalt roads would be welcome here.

Two vehicles and two tents are allowed at each site. All sites are fairly level and not too rocky, and most have excellent shade. There are grassy areas to pitch your tent, but most sites have a large dirt area. There is a vault toilet located on each loop, plus a wheelchair-accessible toilet located near the accessible camping areas along the roadway.

A children's playground is situated near Loop E. There are only two water spigots, one located at Loop C and another at the parking area on the southwestern corner of the lake. The well is treated with chlorine, so filtering is recommended.

The following 13 sites can be reserved May 15–September 15: 3E and 4E on Loop D; 1, 5, 6A, 9, 10, 11, 14, and 17 on Loop E; and 24, 28, and 29 on Loop F.

Annual precipitation averages 19 inches. Summer temperatures rise to around 80°F and can drop into the low 40s many nights. Winter temperatures range from daytime 30s and 40s to single digits at night. This is one of few campgrounds in the mountains of New Mexico that stays open all winter. The park is popular for ice fishing, cross-country skiing, and camping for hunters in early spring or fall.

## :: Key Information

**ADDRESS:** 455 Fenton Lake Rd., Jemez Springs, NM 87025

**OPERATED BY:** New Mexico State Parks

**CONTACT:** 575-829-3630; **www.emnrd.state.nm.us/SPD /fentonlakestatepark.html**

**OPEN:** Year-round, but some sites closed mid-Dec.–mid-March

**SITES:** 36

**SITE AMENITIES:** Parking space, picnic table, pedestal grill, fire ring

**ASSIGNMENT:** First come, first served or reserve at **reserveamerica.com** or 877-664-7787.

**REGISTRATION:** Self-registration on-site without a reservation; with reservation, follow instructions on website and print receipt of reservation for check-in.

**FACILITIES:** Restrooms, vault toilets, picnic shelter, boat ramp

**PARKING:** At each site

**FEE:** $8 primitive, $10 nonelectric, $14 with electric or sewage hookup, $18 with electric and sewage hookups; $5 day-use fee per vehicle

**ELEVATION:** 7,715 feet

**RESTRICTIONS**

■ **Pets:** On 10-foot leash (strictly enforced); take precautionary measures against predators

■ **Fires:** In fire rings only; charcoal grills permitted; check with campground host, Forest Service office, and postings on the camp bulletin board for restrictions.

■ **Alcohol:** At campsites only

■ **Other:** Quiet hours 10 p.m.–8 a.m.; 14-day stay limit

The Fenton Lake State Park rangers are friendly but strict, and the Sandoval County Sheriff's Department patrols with regularity. The New Mexico Department of Fish and Game checks licenses and possession limits frequently.

The fishing here is excellent, and the lake and nearby streams are stocked regularly with rainbow trout by the Seven Springs Fish Hatchery, located 2 miles north on NM 126. You can visit the Seven Springs Fish Hatchery; admission is free, and there is a kids' fishing pond stocked with some large fish. The hatchery also breeds the Rio Grande cutthroat trout and the German brown trout.

Fenton Lake was built in 1946 when a dam was built on Cebolla Creek. The 35-acre lake features a cross-country ski and biathlon trail and wheelchair-accessible fishing platforms. Trout fishing is excellent here, and float tubes, canoes, inflatable rafts, kayaks, and small fishing boats are welcome. Trolling motors are allowed. The 2-mile Hal Baxter Trail loops the park and provides opportunities to view wildlife in its natural habitat.

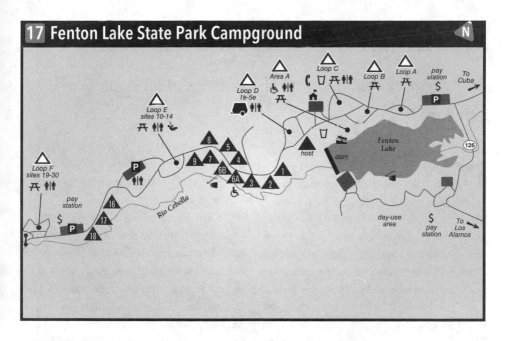

## 17 Fenton Lake State Park Campground

## :: Getting There

From Jemez Springs, drive 11 miles to La Cueva, and turn left (west) onto NM 126. Drive 11 miles to Fenton Lake and turn left at the sign.

**GPS COORDINATES**   N35° 53.133'   W106° 43.477'

**18**

# Clear Creek Campground

*Enjoy remote camping with the benefits of an established campground.*

**I**n the pristine mountains above the town of Cuba, two pretty campgrounds 1 mile apart are a must-stay for the tent camper. Although smaller in size than the other Jemez Wilderness camps in this book, Clear Creek and Rio de las Vacas (see page 75) are for those who want more remote camping with the benefits of an established campground.

Clear Creek is the first campground you reach as you drive up NM 126 from Cuba. The road is now paved past this campground. Previously the traffic along NM 126 would stir gigantic dust clouds that drifted into this camp, but now the air is clear.

There is a tiny stream several inches deep and about a foot wide running through the heart of the campground. The cool water is ideal for foot soaking after a rugged hike. There are no pools to fish here, but the creek adds to the ambience of the place.

The group camping area is set against a hill in the back of the campground. This area has a 40-foot-diameter gazebo and parking separated from the rest of the campground. The group site accommodates

12 tents and can be reserved. Numerous pedestal grills and fire grates are available for the group area.

Clear Creek offers 12 individual campsites, and all are well spaced, grassy, and private. The campground is in a mixed coniferous forest of ponderosa pine, spruce, fir, and a few aspen trees, so most sites are well shaded. Several sites are designated wheelchair accessible. The water system at Clear Creek is provided by a deep well and hand pump, and wheelchair-accessible vault toilets are available.

The Santa Fe National Forest law enforcement officers and the Sandoval County Sheriff's Department frequently patrol the area, and Forest Service employees are always working in this area, so the campground is safe. Cuba Ranger District generally assigns a host either here or at Rio de las Vacas Campground to take care of both camps.

There is no cellular service at the campground. The nearest cellular service and pay telephones are located in Cuba, 11.4 miles away. Cuba has a Saveway Market and a True Value hardware store; both carry camping and fishing supplies and sell New Mexico state fishing licenses. There is also a CC's Paisano Pizzeria and several restaurants if you tire of camp cooking.

Because of the remoteness of this campground and the creek, black bears, mountain lions, bobcats, coyotes, foxes, elk,

## :: Ratings

BEAUTY: ★ ★ ★ ★ ★
PRIVACY: ★ ★ ★ ★
SPACIOUSNESS: ★ ★ ★ ★
QUIET: ★ ★ ★ ★ ★
SECURITY: ★ ★ ★ ★ ★
CLEANLINESS: ★ ★ ★ ★ ★

## :: Key Information

**ADDRESS:** Santa Fe National Forest, Cuba Ranger District, 4 CR 11, Cuba, NM 87103

**OPERATED BY:** U.S. Department of Agriculture

**CONTACT:** 575-289-3264; www.fs.usda.gov/santafe

**OPEN:** Memorial Day–Labor Day

**SITES:** 12, plus group site for up to 60 campers

**SITE AMENITIES:** Parking space, picnic table, pedestal grill, fire ring

**ASSIGNMENT:** First come, first served, except group site can be reserved

**REGISTRATION:** Self-registration on-site

**FACILITIES:** Vault toilets

**PARKING:** At each site

**FEE:** $10, $50 group site

**ELEVATION:** 8,408 feet

**RESTRICTIONS**

■ **Pets:** On 6-foot leash

■ **Fires:** In fire rings only; charcoal grills permitted; check with campground host, Forest Service office, and postings on the camp bulletin board for restrictions.

■ **Alcohol:** At campsites only

■ **Other:** Quiet hours 10 p.m.–8 a.m.; 14-day stay limit

and mule deer are common. Raccoons can wreak havoc here, so please put your food in your vehicle at night. If you read and comply with the bear-alert signs that are posted, you will have no problems with any of the wildlife. Keep pets on a leash at all times and watch children closely. This area of the Jemez Wilderness is open range, meaning cattle are allowed to graze freely all along NM 126. Not all areas are fenced, and cattle are seen walking up and down this road frequently. Please drive carefully. Clear Creek is equipped with a cattle guard at the entrance, and the perimeter is fenced, so rest assured you will not wake up with a 2,000-pound Angus at your camp.

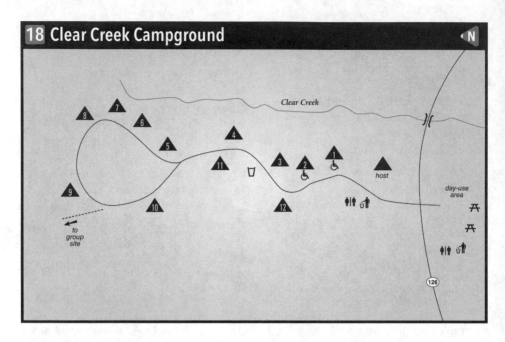

## :: Getting There

From US 550 in Cuba, turn right at the small tourist office and follow NM 126 for 11.4 miles; the campground will be on the left.

**GPS COORDINATES**   N35° 59.778'   W106° 49.618'

# 19

# Rio de las Vacas Campground

*A rushing stream, cascading over boulders with several waist-deep pools, runs the length of the campground.*

**The name** Rio de las Vacas means "river of the cattle" in Spanish, and you'll see plenty of cattle on your way here. Located just 1 mile east of Clear Creek Campground (see page 72), Rio de las Vacas is somewhat larger than Clear Creek, and the campsites are more spacious. The first eight campsites are to the right along the stream. Arrive early if you want one of these spots—they fill up first. However, the streamside sites may pose some inevitable intrusion, as anglers may walk through your camp en route to the stream. From the stream, the road then loops to the left and up a slight incline to the remaining campsites. Eight sites are wheelchair accessible.

There is little road noise here, and quiet hours are respected. The campground is in a mixed coniferous forest, with ponderosa pine, spruce, fir, and a few aspen trees. Because of the forest canopy, most sites are shaded. There are plenty of grassy areas to pitch your tent. The no-odor vault toilets are wheelchair accessible, and pure, sweet-tasting water is provided by a well and hand pump. Raccoons can cause problems here. Please store all coolers and food items in your vehicles. If you read and comply with the posted bear-alert signs, you will have no problems with any of the wildlife.

Santa Fe National Forest law enforcement officers and the Sandoval County Sheriff's Department patrol occasionally. Forest Service employees are always in this area, so security is good. A campground host is assigned either here or at Clear Creek Campground.

Rio de las Vacas is a rushing stream cascading over boulders with several knee- to waist-deep pools—it can be heard throughout the campground. During spring snowmelt and the New Mexico monsoon season, the stream becomes a real torrent, so watch children closely while they play near it. I advise pitching your tent on high ground, as the stream has been known to overrun its banks. Trout anglers have good success here. The headwaters of Rio de las Vacas start at San Gregorio Reservoir, 2 miles to the northwest. Anglers catch several species of trout in the stream: brook, brown, and rainbow. San Gregorio Lake is accessible 1 mile uphill from a marked trail in this campground, and the fishing is generally good there too. As the stream makes its way under the bridge at NM 126, it meanders into an open meadow where you can find

## :: Ratings

BEAUTY: ★ ★ ★ ★ ★
PRIVACY: ★ ★ ★
SPACIOUSNESS: ★ ★ ★ ★
QUIET: ★ ★ ★ ★ ★
SECURITY: ★ ★ ★ ★ ★
CLEANLINESS: ★ ★ ★ ★ ★

## :: Key Information

**ADDRESS:** Santa Fe National Forest, Cuba Ranger District, 4 CR 11, Cuba, NM 87103

**OPERATED BY:** U.S. Department of Agriculture

**CONTACT:** 575-289-3264; www.fs.usda.gov/santafe

**OPEN:** Memorial Day–Labor Day

**SITES:** 15

**SITE AMENITIES:** Parking space, picnic table, fire ring

**ASSIGNMENT:** First come, first served

**REGISTRATION:** Self-registration on-site

**FACILITIES:** Vault toilets

**PARKING:** At each site

**FEE:** $10

**ELEVATION:** 7,880 feet

**RESTRICTIONS**

■ **Pets:** On 6-foot leash; this is black bear country and also home to mountain lions, bobcats, and coyotes, so monitor pets closely.

■ **Fires:** In fire rings only; charcoal grills permitted; check with campground host, Forest Service office, and postings on the camp bulletin board for restrictions.

■ **Alcohol:** At campsites only

■ **Other:** Quiet hours 10 p.m.–8 a.m.; 14-day stay limit

the ruins of an old cabin. This meadow is a lovely place to spend time, and it explodes in color with wildflowers throughout the summer.

There is no cellular service at the campground. The nearest cellular service and pay telephones are located in Cuba, 12.4 miles away. Cuba has a Saveway Market and a True Value hardware store; both carry camping and fishing supplies and sell New Mexico state fishing licenses. There is also a CC's Paisano Pizzeria and several restaurants if you tire of camp cooking.

*Note:* This is open-range country, and cattle abound. You may see cowboys punching cattle along the road. Obey the cowboys' hand signals and instructions; in open-range areas, livestock always have the right of way. Cattle cross NM 126 frequently, so please drive carefully. When hiking, keep your distance from livestock. When walking along NM 126, beware of traffic because four-wheel-drive vehicles, ATVs, and motorcycles speed frequently along this road. There is a cattle guard at the entrance, and the perimeter is fenced, so cattle will not intrude.

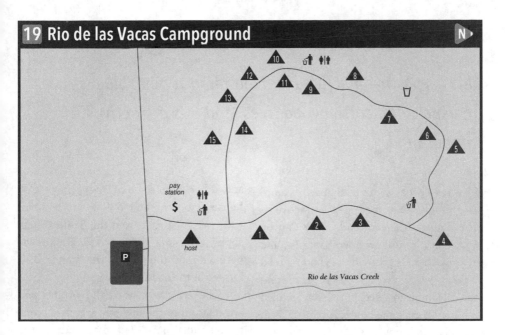

## 19 Rio de las Vacas Campground

## :: Getting There

From US 550 in Cuba, turn right at the small tourist office and follow NM 126 for 12.4 miles; the campground will be on the left.

**GPS COORDINATES**   N35° 59.793'   W106° 48.400'

# 20

# Black Canyon Campground

*This deep canyon is filled with ponderosa pine, blue spruce, fir, aspen, and cottonwood trees, and this attractive little campground.*

**S**anta Fe has some really pretty campgrounds, and the most attractive is Black Canyon Campground. Black Canyon is 7.5 miles from downtown Santa Fe, and the drive there is gorgeous. A winding road works its way from high desert yucca- and sage-filled hills to a deep, lush canyon filled with ponderosa pine, blue spruce, fir, aspen, and tall cottonwood trees.

The Black Canyon is so named because the canyon is steep and deep. While Santa Fe is waking to the early-morning rays of sunlight, the canyon remains dark until the sun crests over the mountain. While the city basks in its sunlight at dusk, the canyon darkens an entire hour before the sun goes down—wonderful for campers who want a few extra winks of sleep.

The entrance to Black Canyon is on the right side of the road. As you enter the campground, you'll find everything new and sparkling-clean. There is a parking lot for the adjoining day-use area, which contains a large gazebo and plenty of space for picnics and other large events. The entrance also houses modern vault toilets and a spigot with water sourced from the Santa Fe city supply. A 1-mile hiking trail circles the perimeter of the camp; the trailhead is located at the back of the campground.

The tent sites begin at the entrance and are adjacent to the highway, which is prone to some road noise, but in all fairness, the traffic becomes very minimal after dark. One large wheelchair-accessible tent site is separated from five other tent sites. These six sites are all reserved for the disabled; they are all walk-in, and the pathways are asphalt to accommodate wheelchairs. A water spigot and varmint-proof trash bin are located halfway down the path. These tent sites are separated by low shrubbery and shaded by the tall conifer forest. All campsites are level and beautifully landscaped, with "designer" cinder block retaining walls and concrete slabs under the picnic table and fire pit area. The fire pits are high quality and ADA-approved with an adjustable cooking grate. The picnic tables are extended on each end for accommodating wheelchair-bound campers. Although some campers may scoff at these concrete pads, I admit they are very easy to keep clean. A small, intermittent stream runs parallel to the tent camping area. The tent sites are spaced apart fairly well.

Past the self-serve pay station, the road runs up the hill past the campground host's

## :: Ratings

BEAUTY: ★ ★ ★ ★ ★
PRIVACY: ★
SPACIOUSNESS: ★
QUIET: ★ ★ ★
SECURITY: ★ ★ ★ ★ ★
CLEANLINESS: ★ ★ ★ ★ ★

## :: Key Information

**ADDRESS:** Santa Fe National Forest, Espanola Ranger District, P.O. Box 3307, Espanola, NM 87113

**OPERATED BY:** U.S. Department of Agriculture

**CONTACT:** 505-753-7331; **www.fs.usda.gov/santafe**

**OPEN:** Mid-April–end of Oct., weather permitting

**SITES:** 36

**SITE AMENITIES:** Parking space, picnic table, lantern hanger, fire ring

**ASSIGNMENT:** Reserve at **reserve america.com** or **recreation.gov** or first come, first served until the date a site is reserved; then you must vacate.

**REGISTRATION:** Self-registration on-site without a reservation; with reservation, follow instructions on website and print receipt of reservation for check-in.

**FACILITIES:** Vault toilets

**PARKING:** At each site

**FEE:** $10 single, $20 double

**ELEVATION:** 8,323 feet

**RESTRICTIONS**

■ **Pets:** On 6-foot leash; take precautionary measures against predators.

■ **Fires:** In fire rings only; charcoal grills permitted; check with campground host, Forest Service office, and postings on the camp bulletin board for restrictions.

■ **Alcohol:** At campsites only

■ **Other:** Quiet hours 10 p.m.–8 a.m.; 14-day stay limit

space, and all the drive-in sites are tightly compacted. Beginning at site 7, all sites are equipped with a concrete pad, gravel tent area, fire ring, lantern pole, and picnic table. Sites 7–10 are designated for the disabled. Sites 23, 26, and 27 are double sites. All five vault toilets are wheelchair accessible, and a water spigot and trash bin are located by each of the five toilet buildings. All facilities are conveniently and equally spaced around the campground. Two commercial-size dumpsters are located in the camp. There is no firewood available here, but you can drive up NM 475 toward the Santa Fe ski basin and find plenty of fallen aspen, fir, and ponderosa pine firewood alongside the road, or you may wish to bring your own.

The camp is beautiful and peaceful in appearance. The rockwork and terracing are well designed and appealing to the eye. If the sites were spaced farther apart, this would be a five-star campground. It is apparent that the architects who designed this campground really haven't spent much time tent camping, and did not take into consideration that a primary requirement for camping is privacy and solitude. For the peace of all who come here, generators are only allowed to be run for 30 minutes every three hours. It's a good policy, but enforcing it is another matter. For maximum peace and quiet, camp during spring or fall and on weekdays if possible to avoid the crowds.

Security is excellent: a host is assigned here, the Forest Service patrols often, and the Santa Fe County Sheriff's Department stops by frequently.

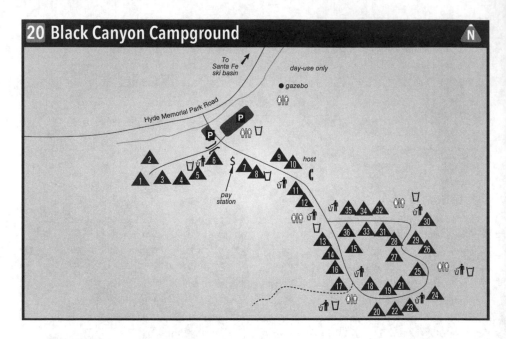

## :: Getting There

From Santa Fe, take Bishop's Lodge Road to Artist Road, which will turn into NM 475 (also known as Hyde Park Road), and travel 7.5 miles to the campground.

**GPS COORDINATES**   N35° 43.683'   W105° 50.398'

# 21

# Field Tract Campground

*The Pecos River runs through it . . . and fills the entire campground with its lovely music.*

**If you** want a little slice of heaven, Field Tract Campground is a great choice. Located off NM 63, just a scant 10 miles north of the historic little town of Pecos, this camp is easy to access. Field Tract is the first developed campground you will come to after entering the Pecos River Wilderness. The Pecos River runs past this campground at a thundering pace, cascading over boulders and filling the entire campground with its lovely music. Despite its location along NM 63, Field Tract is peaceful, and the river drowns out the road noise nicely at most campsites.

Field Tract is a large one-loop campground, with 14 sites. Six of the sites are equipped with Adirondack shelters; these three-sided shelters are constructed of logs and have rock fireplaces. The other campsites are each equipped with a picnic table and fire ring. The tall ponderosa pine trees provide lots of shade, with tall cottonwood trees skirting the river. Tall native grasses abound, almost eliminating the need for a ground pad in many areas. The campsites are not the largest, but there is plenty of space between them, and all are level. Sites 7, 8, 10, and 12 are riverside campsites, and anglers must pass through these sites to access the river.

In the center of the grassy, shaded campground is a large restroom, equipped with sinks and flush toilets. Two other vault toilets are located on the center loop between sites 9 and 11. Three pressurized water spigots are conveniently located across from site 1, between sites 10 and 12, and in the center of the loop by the restroom.

Kids love this campground and have a safe place to pedal bicycles and ride scooters. If they tire of that, the fishing is good here too; the Pecos River is stocked with rainbow trout regularly by the New Mexico Department of Game and Fish, which has numerous fish hatcheries throughout the state. Bird-watchers love it here too, as do photographers. You are welcome to bring bird feeders and enjoy the many species that inhabit this forest. Hummingbirds are thick here and will entertain you for hours, so bring your hummingbird feeder.

Predators live in the area. Although no bears have been spotted at the campground lately, keep a wary eye out just in case. On a starlit night in May, I was startled by one of two German shepherds (belonging to a nearby resident) who run loose in the area; they are shy and will cause you no trouble. The raccoons here are another story: they

## :: Ratings

BEAUTY: ★ ★ ★ ★ ★
PRIVACY: ★ ★ ★ ★
SPACIOUSNESS: ★ ★ ★
QUIET: ★ ★ ★ ★ ★
SECURITY: ★ ★ ★ ★ ★
CLEANLINESS: ★ ★ ★ ★ ★

## :: Key Information

**ADDRESS:** Santa Fe National Forest, Pecos Ranger District, 18 NM 63, Pecos, NM 87552

**OPERATED BY:** U.S. Department of Agriculture

**CONTACT:** 505-757-6121; www.fs.usda.gov/santafe

**OPEN:** Mid-May–mid-Sept.

**SITES:** 14

**SITE AMENITIES:** Parking space, picnic table, fire ring; 6 sites equipped with Adirondack shelters

**ASSIGNMENT:** First come, first served

**REGISTRATION:** Self-registration on-site

**FACILITIES:** 2 vault toilets, 1 flush toilet; bring water

**PARKING:** At each site

**FEE:** $8

**ELEVATION:** 7,429 feet

**RESTRICTIONS**

■ **Pets:** On 6-foot leash; take precautionary measures against predators

■ **Fires:** In fire rings only; charcoal grills permitted; check with campground host, Forest Service office, and postings on the camp bulletin board for restrictions.

■ **Alcohol:** At campsites only

■ **Other:** Quiet hours 10 p.m.–8 a.m.; 14-day stay limit

are plentiful and will rob you blind, so pack away your food at night.

Security here is excellent; San Miguel County Sheriff's Department, Forest Service officers, and New Mexico Department of Game and Fish wardens patrol this area constantly. Have your fishing license available because the fishing laws here are strictly enforced. The campground host usually sells firewood, but any nearby forest road will provide gathering spots for all the wood you need.

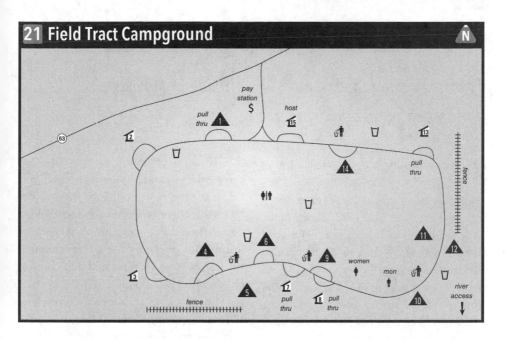

## :: Getting There

From Pecos, travel 10 miles north on NM 63, and the campground is on the right.

**GPS COORDINATES**   N35° 41.240'   W105° 41.660'

# Iron Gate Campground

*This gem is perched on a mountainside of spruce, fir, ponderosa pine, and aspen trees.*

**A**fter enduring the gut-wrenching drive of 4.3 miles up Pecos's bumpy Forest Service Road 223, you will enjoy the quiet camping experience at Iron Gate Campground. This is a one-loop campground, with good spacing between sites, and all the shaded sites are fairly private. Sites 7 and 8 at the end of the loop are walk-in sites, less than 50 feet from the road. Sites 1, 3, 11, 12, 13, and 14 are in the open with no shade, but the remaining sites are under tree cover. The entire camp has deep grass, with wildflowers blooming.

There are four horse corrals. One vault toilet is located at the entrance, and a second is located off the end loop. Two varmint-proof trash bins are located near the toilets. If these bins are full, you must pack out your trash. There is no water, so pack in enough to douse your fire completely. An axe and shovel are mandatory at these remote camps, and I recommend a lawn rake as well. There is plenty of firewood along the road outside of camp, especially downed aspen trees. If aspen wood is dry, it makes an excellent campfire.

## :: Ratings

BEAUTY: ★ ★ ★ ★ ★
PRIVACY: ★ ★ ★ ★
SPACIOUSNESS: ★ ★ ★ ★ ★
QUIET: ★ ★ ★ ★ ★
SECURITY: ★ ★
CLEANLINESS: ★ ★ ★ ★ ★

There is plenty of parking, and the camp road is gravel. There isn't much traffic, so for the most part, your site will not be dusty. There is no host, but the Forest Service keeps an eye on this place. Because it is remote, predatory animals can frequent this camp. Keep this in mind and monitor children and pets closely.

Iron Gate sits at more than 9,200 feet, so it gets quite cold here at night; be sure to pack a warm sleeping bag. Expect lows in the low 40°F range most nights, even in summer. Daytime temperatures rarely exceed 80°F. When it rains, the runoff is good, but stake your tent on high ground. Bring a tarp to stretch over the picnic table. High elevations here in the Pecos Wilderness are susceptible to torrential downpours. Being on the side of a mountain poses issues with lightning strikes as well, so be ready to take cover.

Trail 250 begins at the end of the loop and travels 10 miles over elevations ranging from 9,200 to 11,400 feet. This trail is moderate to difficult, and usage is light to moderate. Equestrians are welcome on Trail 250 too.

*Note:* Because of the Tres Lagunas Fire, flooding on NM 63 is a strong possibility during the rainy season. The Forest Service may close or deny access to this campground, or access to NM 63, when flooding is a threat. FR 223 is an undeveloped, steep road with deep ruts; four-wheel-drive vehicles are strongly recommended, especially during inclement weather. It would be unwise to attempt this road with an RV.

## :: Key Information

**ADDRESS:** Santa Fe National Forest, Pecos Ranger District, 18 NM 63, Pecos, NM 87552

**OPERATED BY:** U.S. Department of Agriculture

**CONTACT:** 505-757-6121; www.fs.usda.gov/santafe

**OPEN:** May 1–Oct. 1, weather permitting

**SITES:** 14

**SITE AMENITIES:** Parking space, picnic table, fire ring

**ASSIGNMENT:** First come, first served

**REGISTRATION:** Self-registration on-site

**FACILITIES:** Vault toilets, horse corrals; bring water.

**PARKING:** At each site

**FEE:** $4 per night per vehicle

**ELEVATION:** 9,243 feet

**RESTRICTIONS**

■ **Pets:** On 6-foot leash

■ **Fires:** In fire rings only; charcoal grills permitted; check with campground host, Forest Service office, and postings on the camp bulletin board for restrictions.

■ **Alcohol:** At campsites only

■ **Other:** Quiet hours 10 p.m.–8 a.m.; 14-day stay limit; max 3 cars per site

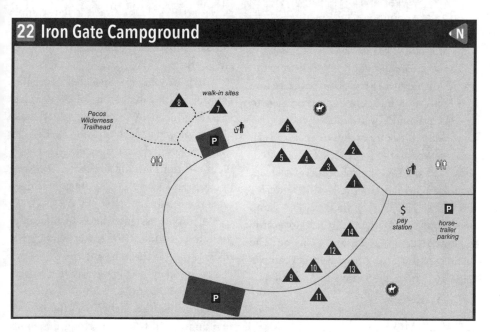

## :: Getting There

From Cowles, drive 0.75 mile south on NM 63 to FR 223. The road is well marked, so follow signs to campground. Drive slowly due to dust, and respect the homeowners along this road. Do not trespass on private property.

**GPS COORDINATES**   N35° 50.348'   W105° 37.302'

# 23

# Jack's Creek Campground

*With breathtaking mountain vistas and deep, lush forests, Jack's Creek is worthy of its five-star rating.*

**I**f there is a campground worthy of a five-star rating, Jack's Creek has to be it. It is an absolute diamond. Jack's Creek is the last campground you come to in the Pecos Wilderness, and it's the second highest in elevation, at almost 9,000 feet, of all the Pecos campgrounds. During my visit in late June, I heard woodpeckers working in the forests.

The campground is surrounded by a lush grassy forest of tall, mature aspen, ponderosa pine, fir, and spruce trees, and the mountain vistas are breathtaking—12,622-foot Santa Fe Baldy is visible from the camp, with snowfields visible above tree line elevations well into July. You would have to travel far to find a prettier location.

Jack's Creek is easily accessible, with paved roads all the way to the campground. However, the road hairpins and gets steep, and there are no guardrails, so it's not for drivers with a fear of heights. The camp is separated into three distinct areas: the equestrian camp, two group camps, and the main camping area. The equestrian camp is separated from the main camp by its own road. The two group camps—Group A and Group B—are by reservation only and cost $50 per night.

The campsites here are extremely large and well spaced for privacy. Sites on the inside of the loop have little shade but better grass. Sites on the outer loops have tall, shady conifers and aspens but lack grass. All sites are level and can accommodate tents as well as RVs. Jack's Creek is tent-camper friendly. Generator run times are restricted to 30 minutes every 3 hours and prohibited after dark.

All restrooms are wheelchair accessible, equipped with composting toilets, and kept sparkling clean. A water spigot and trash bin are located at each restroom, with other water spigots and trash bins placed at convenient locations around the camp. The water is clean and sweet-tasting, but filtering is recommended.

A host is assigned here, so the campground is secure. The Forest Service frequently patrols the area, and the equestrian campground is a staging area for search-and-rescue operations.

*Note:* Because of the Tres Lagunas Fire, flooding on NM 63 is a strong possibility during the rainy season. The Forest Service may close or deny access to this campground, or access to NM 63, when flooding is a threat.

## :: Ratings

BEAUTY: ★ ★ ★ ★ ★
PRIVACY: ★ ★ ★
SPACIOUSNESS: ★ ★ ★ ★ ★
QUIET: ★ ★ ★ ★ ★
SECURITY: ★ ★ ★ ★
CLEANLINESS: ★ ★ ★ ★ ★

## :: Key Information

**ADDRESS:** Santa Fe National Forest, Pecos Ranger District, 18 NM 63, Pecos, NM 87552

**OPERATED BY:** U.S. Department of Agriculture

**CONTACT:** 505-757-6121; **www.fs.usda.gov/santafe**

**OPEN:** Memorial Day–Labor Day

**SITES:** 38

**SITE AMENITIES:** Parking space, picnic table, fire ring

**ASSIGNMENT:** First come, first served

**REGISTRATION:** Self-registration on-site

**FACILITIES:** Vault toilets

**PARKING:** At each site

**FEE:** $10

**ELEVATION:** 8,936 feet

**RESTRICTIONS**

■ **Pets:** On 6-foot leash; take precautionary measures against predators.

■ **Fires:** In fire rings only; charcoal grills permitted; check with campground host, Forest Service office, and postings on the camp bulletin board for restrictions.

■ **Alcohol:** At campsites only

■ **Other:** Quiet hours 10 p.m.–8 a.m.; 14-day stay limit

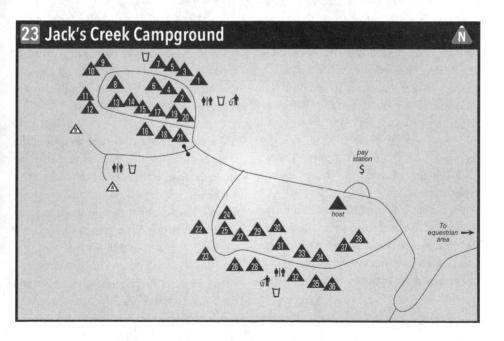

**23 Jack's Creek Campground**

## :: Getting There

Follow NM 63 to Cowles; at the junction, follow Forest Service Road 555 for 3.4 miles to the campground.

**GPS COORDINATES**   N35° 50.318'   W105° 39.317'

# 24

# Villanueva State Park

*A delightful place set in a canyon of brilliant sandstone cliffs.*

**S**ituated in a lush, fertile valley surrounded by mountains, mesas, and sheer dramatic cliffs, Villanueva Sate Park is a delightful place with a slow, relaxed pace that takes you back to the 1800s. The park was named after the town of Villanueva, which you will pass through on your way to the park.

Villanueva State Park can be accessed from two directions. Coming from Santa Fe or Las Vegas, New Mexico, Villanueva is 12 miles south of the I-25 exit. From Albuquerque, the drive from I-40 north on NM 3 is the most scenic, as you make the breathtaking descent into this pretty green valley. The name Villanueva means "new village" in Spanish. The town was established in 1890, and several old buildings and crumbling adobes seem to contradict the town's name. Two small general stores provide basic groceries but no camping supplies. The zip code directory of the entire valley lists only 217 addresses.

Villanueva State Park was established in 1967 and is one of the most modern facilities in the New Mexico state park system. The park receives more than 48,000 visitors per year, and the majority of campers arrive over the weekends between May and September. Gate hours are 7 a.m.–9 p.m. daily. The rangers are helpful and friendly, and they patrol often, as does the San Miguel County Sheriff's Department. The visitor center offers valuable information and several wildlife displays.

The park itself is set in a canyon of 500-foot-high red-and-yellow sandstone cliffs. With plenty of trees, you will have no trouble finding shade; plus the canyon walls block the sun in the mornings and afternoons. The campground altitude averages 5,800 feet, and it gets quite chilly in early spring or late fall. In summer, the shady canyon is cooler than the open valley, where temperatures reach the high 90s.

The campground is divided into several areas; the RV area is separated from the nonelectric campsites. Several tent sites are along the road at the park entrance, but they are small and afford no privacy; however, they do have adequate shade and a modern vault toilet with a water spigot. The self-pay station is across from these sites.

The RV area is across the road from the visitor center. A large group picnic area and the comfort stations are located there. The comfort stations are equipped with showers and kept spotlessly clean.

Past the group picnic shelter to the right are campsites located on both sides of the road. The best sites are to the right, alongside the Pecos River. The soil at these riverside sites is a mix of sand and sparse grasses, making this area a good choice for tent

## :: Ratings

BEAUTY: ★ ★ ★ ★ ★
PRIVACY: ★ ★ ★ ★
SPACIOUSNESS: ★ ★ ★ ★
QUIET: ★ ★ ★ ★
SECURITY: ★ ★ ★ ★ ★
CLEANLINESS: ★ ★ ★ ★ ★

## :: Key Information

**ADDRESS:** 135 Dodge Rd., Villanueva, NM 87583

**OPERATED BY:** New Mexico State Parks

**CONTACT:** 575-421-2957; **www.emnrd .state.nm.us/SPD/villanuevastatepark .html**

**OPEN:** April 1–Sept. 30

**SITES:** 33

**SITE AMENITIES:** Parking space, picnic table, fire ring

**ASSIGNMENT:** First come, first served or reserve at **reserveamerica.com** or 877-664-7787.

**REGISTRATION:** Self-registration on-site without a reservation; with reservation, follow instructions on website and print receipt of reservation for check-in.

**FACILITIES:** Vault toilets, restrooms, showers, visitor center, playground, dump station

**PARKING:** At each site

**FEE:** $8 primitive, $10 nonelectric, $14 with electric or sewage hookup, $18 with electric and sewage hookups; $5 day-use fee per vehicle

**ELEVATION:** 5,749 feet

**RESTRICTIONS**

■ **Pets:** On 10-foot leash; this is black bear country and also home to mountain lions, bobcats, coyotes, and rattlesnakes, so monitor pets closely.

■ **Fires:** In fire rings only; charcoal grills permitted; check with campground host, Forest Service office, and postings on the camp bulletin board for restrictions.

■ **Alcohol:** At campsites only

■ **Other:** Quiet hours 10 p.m.–8 a.m.; 14-day stay limit

camping. The riverside area is quite shady, with a mix of Rio Grande cottonwood, coyote willow, Chinese elm, and mature juniper and piñon trees. These trees do a nice job of curtaining you from other campsites; you will appreciate the privacy. Each of the sites along the river has a covered shelter.

El Cerro camping area is up the hill and to the left; it holds 10 campsites with several shelters and one modern vault toilet. The ground is quite rocky here, so bring a thick ground pad. Although you will not have the ambience of a riverside campground, you will be up on a hill with a great view of most of the park, the river, and the cliffs.

Past the riverside campsites, there is a large picnic area and a modern playground. Children love Villanueva because there are safe places to play and nice areas for bicycle rides. The Pecos River runs year-round and has a strong current during the spring snowmelt or during the monsoon season. Canoeing, tubing, rafting, and swimming in the Pecos River are popular summer activities, but there is no lifeguard on duty. Before getting into the river, check with a ranger for any hazards you may encounter, and by all means be careful. PFDs and life vests are mandatory equipment while you are on the river.

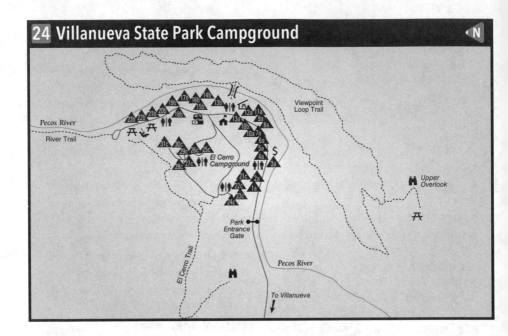

## :: Getting There

*From Santa Fe:* Take I-25 to Exit 363 and follow NM 3 south for 12 miles through the town of Villanueva; follow signs to the park.

*From Albuquerque:* Take I-40 to Exit 230 and follow NM 3 north for 20 miles through the town of Villanueva; follow signs to the park.

**GPS COORDINATES**   N35° 15.833'   W105° 20.417'

# 25

# Cochiti Lake Campgrounds

*Cochiti provides an ideal desert-lake camping experience.*

**C**ochiti Lake Campgrounds offer ideal desert-lake camping experiences for many reasons. Cochiti Dam is the 11th largest in the United States, using 65 million cubic feet of earth and rock. Construction took 10 years and was completed in 1975 at a cost of $94.4 million. There are two campgrounds, the main campground at Cochiti Lake headquarters and Tetilla Peak Campground on the opposite side of the lake. Shoreline camping is not available at either campground.

The original main Cochiti campground is divided into three loops: Chamisa, Juniper, and Apache Plume. The Chamisa Loop has 34 tent sites with 17 covered shelters and plenty of parking. Chamisa has two vault toilets, and the restroom with the shower is a short walk up the hill from site 4. All restrooms are spotless. Juniper and piñon trees, along with bushes, ensure sites are semi-private. Apache Plume Loop stays closed unless it's reserved by a group or needed as an overflow area. This loop has 21 sites, with covered shelters, picnic tables, and pedestal grills at each site. No restrooms or water spigots are available within this loop.

## :: Ratings

BEAUTY: ★ ★ ★
PRIVACY: ★ ★
SPACIOUSNESS: ★ ★
QUIET: ★ ★ ★ ★ ★
SECURITY: ★ ★ ★ ★ ★
CLEANLINESS: ★ ★ ★ ★ ★

Juniper Campground is the RV area. Each site has a water spigot and 30- or 50-amp electrical hookups.

In 2012, three new campground loops were built at Cochiti Lake: Buffalo Grove, Elk Run, and Ringtail Cat. These loops are located on the east side of the road as you are heading south toward the boat ramp and are designed with RV campers in mind. (With that said, the original Chamisa Loop is an excellent tent area and is not set up for RVs.) The new nonelectric sites are intended to attract both tent and RV campers, but with no electricity, the tent campers at these new loops will be listening to generators running at all hours. All the new sites have a sun shelter, picnic table, lantern post, tent pad filled with pea gravel, and grill. There are no fire pits because ground fires are prohibited here. Buffalo Grove Loop has 16 RV sites, with water and electricity at each site. Elk Run Loop has 16 RV/tent sites, no electricity, and three water spigots evenly spaced in the loop. Ringtail Cat Loop has 12 RV/tent sites, no electricity, and three water spigots evenly spaced in the loop. All of these new loops have their own fully equipped restroom with warm-water showers, and all sites here have elongated parking pads for RVs or boat trailers.

Tetilla Peak Campground is divided into two loops for RVs with a total of 44 sites and a tent area with 10 sites. There are three restrooms, and five water spigots are distributed at equal distances throughout the campground.

## :: Key Information

**ADDRESS:** Cochiti Lake Office, 82 Dam Crest Rd., Pena Blanca, NM 87041

**OPERATED BY:** United States Army Corps of Engineers, Albuquerque District

**CONTACT:** 505-465-0307; **www.spa .usace.army.mil/Missions/CivilWorks /Recreation/CochitiLake.aspx**

**OPEN:** *Main campground* year-round (Chamisa Loop closed in winter); *Tetilla Peak* April 1–Oct. 31

**SITES:** *Main campground* 129; *Tetilla Peak* 54

**SITE AMENITIES:** Parking space, picnic table, pedestal charcoal grill; many have covered shelters.

**ASSIGNMENT:** Reserve at **reserve america.com** or **recreation.gov** or first come, first served.

**REGISTRATION:** At office; if office unattended, self-registration on-site without a reservation; with reservation, follow instructions on website and print receipt of reservation for check-in.

**FACILITIES:** Restrooms, showers, vault toilets, visitor center, boat ramps, dump stations

**PARKING:** At each site

**FEE:** $12 tent site (max 2 tents and 1 vehicle per site); $20 full hookup

**ELEVATION:** 5,400–5500 feet

**RESTRICTIONS**

■ **Pets:** On leash at all times (strictly enforced); not allowed at swimming beaches

■ **Fires:** No ground fires whatsoever; charcoal or wood fires in pedestal grills except during high winds or when Stage II fire restrictions are in effect; propane grills permitted during Stage II fire restrictions

■ **Alcohol:** Not permitted

■ **Other:** Quiet Hours 10 p.m.–8 a.m.; 14-day stay limit; gates locked 10 p.m.– 6 a.m. every night—gate combination code issued at check-in

Cochiti Lake has a beautiful sand swimming beach with covered sun shelters, but no lifeguard is present. I have paddled my raft all over this clean, fun lake. The lake is a no-wake lake, and it's strictly enforced. Mandatory U.S. Coast Guard–approved life vests are required on the lake everywhere except the swimming beach.

Within a 6-mile drive is the Kasha-Katuwe Tent Rocks National Monument, managed by the Bureau of Land Management.

This is a must-see for any Cochiti camper. Take NM 22 to the base of the dam, turn west onto Cochiti Reservation Road 84, and follow the sign to Forest Service Road 266 and the small roadway office. Fee is $5 per day. You'll find 3 miles of easy-to-moderate hiking trails at Tent Rocks. Be sure to hike the canyon trail, as the canyon is very narrow and incredible for photographers and artists. While on American Indian tribal land, be respectful and obey all laws.

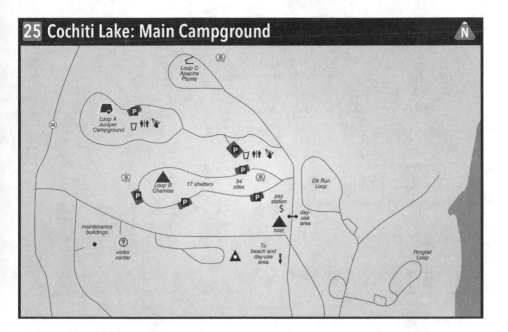

**25** Cochiti Lake: Main Campground

## :: Getting There

### MAIN CAMPGROUND

From I-25, take Exit 264 and drive northwest on NM 22 for 12 miles to Cochiti Dam entrance.

### TETILLA PEAK CAMPGROUND *(see map next page)*

From I-25, take Exit 264 and drive northwest on NM 22 for 8 miles; follow NM 16 for 10 miles to the Tetilla Peak entrance.

### GPS COORDINATES

**Main Campground**   N35° 38.547'   W106° 19.525'

**Tetilla Peak Campground**   N35° 38.737'   W106° 18.403'

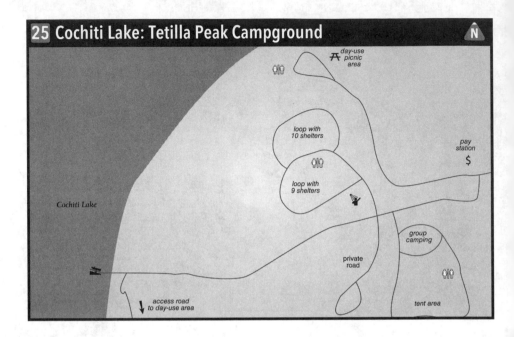

**25** Cochiti Lake: Tetilla Peak Campground

N

day-use picnic area

loop with 10 shelters

loop with 9 shelters

pay station

$

group camping

Cochiti Lake

private road

tent area

access road to day-use area

# Southeastern New Mexico

# 26

# Manzano Mountains State Park

*Manzano is one of the loveliest of all New Mexico state parks.*

**M**anzano Mountains State Park is located just 51 miles from the city limits of Albuquerque. The entire drive south on NM 337 is beautiful. This state park was established in 1978 and encompasses 160 acres.

On November 19, 2007, the Ojo Peak Fire started south of Red Canyon Campground, burning more than 7,500 acres. On the night of Thanksgiving, Mother Nature sent several inches of snow into the area, and the fire stopped just west of the park, sparing Manzano Mountains State Park.

Manzano is a must for tent campers, though you will find that several RVs are always present in the main loop. There are 23 developed sites in the main loop and 31 primitive sites in the group area. The group area can be opened to tent campers as an overflow area when all of the loop spots are filled. I've camped in the group area numerous times, setting up my tent in the shade of the juniper and piñon trees. There is a beautiful gazebo for group camping, and you'll appreciate it if a thunderstorm hits. The area has several trash bins, numerous fire rings, and picnic tables scattered around the various sites.

## :: Ratings

BEAUTY: ★ ★ ★ ★ ★
PRIVACY: ★ ★ ★ ★
SPACIOUSNESS: ★ ★ ★ ★
QUIET: ★ ★ ★ ★ ★
SECURITY: ★ ★ ★ ★ ★
CLEANLINESS: ★ ★ ★ ★ ★

The water system is pressurized, and the state park regularly checks and treats the water. The restrooms are sparkling clean with flush toilets and sinks but no showers.

This camp is very secure. A campground manager lives on-site, and the New Mexico Parks Department and the Torrance County Sheriff's Department patrol regularly. The park office is open on weekends and loans reading material on the plants and animals endemic to the area. You can also obtain a list of bird species that are native to the park. Steller's jays and Abert's squirrels are quite entertaining and easy to photograph at the feeders in front of the park office. Bring your hummingbird feeder; you will be happy you did. The Manzano Mountains are a great place to be if you love birds. It is a main migratory flyway, and many raptors follow the waterfowl back and forth.

The forest here is a mixture of ponderosa pine, piñon, Gambel oak, Emory oak, and alligator juniper trees. The alligator juniper is named for the checkered pattern on the bark of older trees, which resembles an alligator's hide. If you hike back into the forest, there are plenty of piñon nuts you can gather for a healthy camp snack. Several easy nature trails meander through the park.

The name Manzano means "apple tree" in Spanish, but there are no apple trees here. The apple trees in the Manzano Mountains were planted by Spanish missionaries throughout this area in the 1800s. The remaining trees are believed to be the oldest living apple trees in the United States.

## :: Key Information

**ADDRESS:** Manzano Mountains State Park, Mile Marker 3 NM 131, Mountainair, NM 87036

**OPERATED BY:** New Mexico State Parks

**CONTACT:** 505-344-7240; **www.emnrd .state.nm.us/SPD/manzanomountains statepark.html**

**OPEN:** April 1–Nov. 1

**SITES:** 23 developed sites; 31 primitive sites

**SITE AMENITIES:** Parking space, picnic table, fire ring; developed sites have water and sewer; 9 with electricity

**ASSIGNMENT:** First come, first served or reserve at **reserveamerica.com** or 877-664-7787.

**REGISTRATION:** Self-registration on-site without a reservation; with reservation, follow instructions on website and print receipt of reservation for check-in.

**FACILITIES:** Restrooms, visitor center

**PARKING:** At each site

**FEE:** $8 primitive, $10 nonelectric, $14 with electric and sewage hookup

**ELEVATION:** 7,259 feet

**RESTRICTIONS**

■ **Pets:** On 6-foot leash

■ **Fires:** In fire rings only; charcoal grills permitted

■ **Alcohol:** At campsites only

■ **Other:** Quiet hours 10 p.m.–8 a.m.; 14-day stay limit; gate hours 7:30 a.m.– sunset

There is no firewood at this campground—it has been picked clean—but if you drive into the forest west on Forest Service Road 253, you will find plenty of firewood. There is a wood yard on the main highway at the state park turnoff road that sells alligator juniper; it is great for burning and has a beautiful scent.

Be prepared to cold-camp during the dry seasons. The Manzano Mountains get far less precipitation (only 14.2 inches per year) than the mountains in Northern New Mexico. When fire restrictions go into effect in the adjacent Cibola National Forest, this state park takes the same action. Every year Stage II fire restrictions are a reality here, but don't let that discourage you from camping here.

The Manzano Mountains are substantially warmer than the mountains to the north. Because of this, all of the campgrounds open in April. I was delighted to wake up to a beautiful 6-inch snowfall here in late April. It melted fast, and the mercury rose to 60°F by noon.

The Manzano Tiendita on Forest Service Road 55 does not carry many camping supplies, but it does offer adequate groceries and ice, and the prices are reasonable. A town named Punte de Agua is 5 miles south of Manzano, and the Quarai Ruins, part of the Salinas Pueblo Missions National Monument, are just 1 mile west of Punte de Agua. The Tiwa Pueblo here was already in existence in 1529 when Spanish explorer Juan de Onate discovered it in 1598. The mission was established in 1629. Other nearby attractions include numerous hiking trails and the Tajique/Torreon horseshoe drive down FR 55. Please inquire at the park office for more information.

## 26 Manzano Mountains State Park Campground

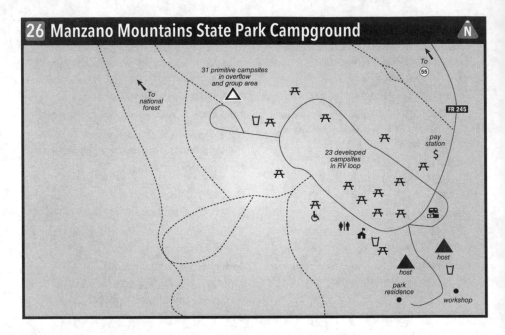

## :: Getting There

From NM 337 in Manzano, turn right at the Manzano Mountains State Park sign, following FR 245 for 3 miles. When the asphalt road turns to the right, follow the signs and the gravel road straight, and Manzano is just ahead at the top of the hill.

**GPS COORDINATES**   N34° 36.196'   W106° 21.685'

# 27

# Red Canyon Campground

*Red Canyon is semiremote and beautiful.*

**R**ed Canyon Campground is situated in a forest of ponderosa pine, with scattered fir, spruce, Gambel oak, and aspen trees. I have been here dozens of times and never seen this campground full. The real attraction to this lovely setting is that it's underused. The dirt road to Red Canyon has a few bumpy spots but is well maintained.

Due to extreme drought conditions, Red Canyon nearly became a victim of a wildfire. On November 19, 2007, the Ojo Peak Fire started south of Red Canyon, burning more than 7,500 acres. Fire damage is apparent all around, but the campground was spared. To get there you will need to drive through the Ojo Peak Fire burn scar.

The campground is divided into two camps. Driving to your right uphill, you'll find the equestrian camp with parking for trailers and corrals for horses. The lower camp, 50 yards farther to the south, is for tent campers and RVs. There are 18 sites at the equestrian camp and 20 sites at the lower camp. There is usually an RV or two here, but they're limited to 22 feet. All sites provide liberal shade. Red Canyon is a good choice if you're looking for serenity

## :: Ratings

BEAUTY: ★ ★ ★ ★ ★
PRIVACY: ★ ★ ★ ★ ★
SPACIOUSNESS: ★ ★ ★ ★
QUIET: ★ ★ ★ ★ ★
SECURITY: ★
CLEANLINESS: ★ ★ ★ ★ ★

and peace. Several easy-to-moderate hiking trails are here, and the trail information is posted right at the trailhead in the campground.

There is no water available at the camp, but you might be able to fill up at Manzano Mountains State Park, 3 miles away. The pit toilets are in good condition and clean. There is no campground host assigned here. There may be an occasional patrol by the Forest Service or the Torrance County Sheriff's Department, but don't count on much security.

This campground is protected by mountains on two sides and a tall canopy of ponderosa pines. When it gets windy, you are well protected. When it rains, a mud bog forms in the center of the campground because of poor drainage. Select a site on the outside of the loops where the runoff is better. There is plenty of firewood. As in all national forests, it is mandatory to carry a shovel and axe. Be careful with your campfire, because the only water available is what you carry in.

Due to its remote location, Red Canyon sees black bears, mountain lions, bobcats, coyotes, and raccoons. There are no bear-proof food boxes here, so keep your food in your vehicle. The trash bins are bear-proof. Read and comply with the bear-alert postings and you should be safe. Occasionally there is stagnant water in the streambed, so mosquitoes might be a problem. Deer and elk droppings are also found frequently here, so beware of deer ticks.

The Manzano Tiendita on Forest Service Road 55 does not carry many camping

## :: Key Information

**ADDRESS:** Cibola National Forest, Mountainair Ranger District, P.O. Box 69, Mountainair, NM 87036

**OPERATED BY:** U.S. Department of Agriculture

**CONTACT:** 505-847-2990; www.fs.usda.gov/cibola

**OPEN:** Memorial Day–Labor Day

**SITES:** 38

**SITE AMENITIES:** Parking space, picnic table, fire ring

**ASSIGNMENT:** First come, first served

**REGISTRATION:** Self-registration on-site

**FACILITIES:** Vault toilets, horse corrals; bring water.

**PARKING:** At each site

**FEE:** $7

**ELEVATION:** 7,714 feet

**RESTRICTIONS**

■ **Pets:** On 6-foot leash; this is black bear country and also home to mountain lions, bobcats, and coyotes, so monitor pets closely.

■ **Fires:** In fire rings only; charcoal grills permitted; check with the Forest Service office and postings on the camp bulletin board for restrictions.

■ **Alcohol:** At campsites only

■ **Other:** Quiet hours 10 p.m.–8 a.m.; 14-day stay limit

supplies, but it does offer adequate groceries and ice, the prices are reasonable, and the owners are friendly. A town named Punte de Agua is 5 miles south of Manzano. There is a small park there with a gazebo and a windmill pressurizing the well, but the quality of the water is unknown. Don't miss the Quarai Ruins, part of the Salinas Pueblo Missions National Monument, just 12 miles from the campground. The Tiwa Pueblo here was already in existence in 1529 when Spanish explorer Juan de Onate discovered it in 1598. The mission was established in 1629. The Tajique/Torreon horseshoe drive is an enjoyable side trip on FR 55 in Torreon.

## :: Getting There

From the town of Manzano, follow the road signs leading to Manzano Mountains State Park. This is FR 253. Stay on FR 253 for 3 miles until you arrive at the Manzano Mountains State Park entrance sign. At this three-way intersection, the road turns 90 degrees. Turn right and stay on this road. From the three-way intersection, it is another 3 miles to the entrances. The road forks to the right and up the hill to the equestrian camp. The main campground entrance is only 50 yards straight ahead.

**GPS COORDINATES**　N34° 36.967'　W106° 24.200'

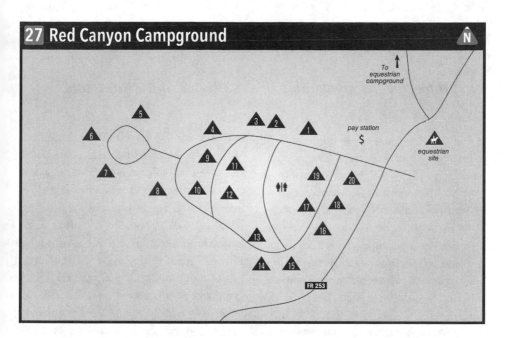

**27** **Red Canyon Campground**

To equestrian campground

pay station
$

equestrian site

5
6
7
4
3
2
1
9
11
8
10
12
19
20
17
18
16
13
14
15

FR 253

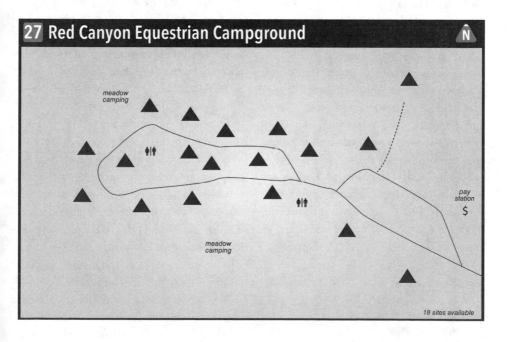

**27** **Red Canyon Equestrian Campground**

meadow camping

pay station
$

meadow camping

18 sites available

# 28

# Fourth of July Campground

*This tent camper's paradise offers plenty of hiking trails.*

**I**f **ever** there was a paradise for tent campers, Fourth of July Campground has to be it. The sign at the entrance reads: "RV Camping at Red Canyon Campground," so you won't see any big rigs here. Most parking places are just large enough for a car. Pop-up campers are welcome, but it would be a tight squeeze getting a pop-up camper and a tow vehicle into one space. The campground host site is set up at the entrance of the campground and has electricity. The host has the only hard-sided RV allowed in the camp.

Camping spots are well shaded in a forest of ponderosa pine, spruce, alligator juniper, piñon, big-toothed maple, aspen, and Gambel oak trees. This campground is well designed for tents. Although some sites are spaced closely together, most areas provide enough space to afford privacy, and there is plenty of room to set your tent back and away from others. The two camping loops are named Gallo and Masca. Both loops have two modern cinderblock vault toilets with solar-powered lighting and bear-proof trash bins. Gallo has smaller campsites, so check Masca first if you want a roomier area.

## :: Ratings

BEAUTY: ★ ★ ★ ★ ★
PRIVACY: ★ ★ ★
SPACIOUSNESS: ★ ★ ★
QUIET: ★ ★ ★
SECURITY: ★ ★ ★ ★ ★
CLEANLINESS: ★ ★ ★ ★ ★

Gallo curves off to the left with 16 single sites. Masca Loop has five single sites, one double site with two tables and two fire rings, and one triple site with three tables and three fire rings. All single sites have a fire ring, table, and parking spot. Both loops are fairly long; a round-trip bicycle ride is 0.75 mile. This is a great campground for kids, with lots of room to play. A campground host is assigned here from Memorial Day through Labor day, and the Forest Service and Torrance County Sheriff's Department frequently patrol the area, so this campground is very secure.

Fortunately, Fourth of July Campground and the area surrounding it were not affected by the Trigo Fire. You can see the tremendous damage the fire had upon the forests as you drive up Forest Service Road 55. A few miles past Tajique Campground, the forest thickens and is as beautiful as always. FR 55 is well maintained because there are areas adjacent to the forest that are privately owned. The entire 17-mile length of FR 55 is a magnificently beautiful drive despite the Trigo Fire. That said, however, flash flooding on FR 55 can be a concern.

Three moderate trails are located within the campground and range from 0.8 mile to 3.5 miles in length. There is a parking lot specifically for hikers at the campground entrance. Trail maps are available at the pay station. Day-use and hiking fees are $5 per day. Incidentally, this is a great place to launch backpacking trips. No off-road vehicles are allowed on the trails.

# :: Key Information

**ADDRESS:** Cibola National Forest, Mountainair Ranger District, P.O. Box 69, Mountainair, NM 87036

**OPERATED BY:** U.S. Department of Agriculture

**CONTACT:** 505-847-2990; www.fs.usda.gov/cibola

**OPEN:** April–Oct., depending on weather

**SITES:** 23

**SITE AMENITIES:** Parking space, picnic table, fire ring

**ASSIGNMENT:** First come, first served

**REGISTRATION:** Self-registration on-site

**FACILITIES:** Restrooms; bring water.

**PARKING:** At each site

**FEE:** $7

**ELEVATION:** 7,505 feet

**RESTRICTIONS**

■ **Pets:** On 6-foot leash; take precautionary measures against predators.

■ **Fires:** In fire rings only; charcoal grills permitted; check with campground host, Forest Service office, and postings on the camp bulletin board for restrictions.

■ **Alcohol:** At campsites only

■ **Other:** Quiet hours 10 p.m.–8 a.m.; 14-day stay limit

The campground usually opens in April and may stay open as late as November, weather permitting. Camping here before Memorial Day and after Labor Day is awesome. It gets cool at night, sometimes reaching the low 40s. Black bears, mountain lions, bobcats, and coyotes are common, so obey the posted alerts. Occasional rattlesnakes have been spotted here, so watch your kids and pets closely.

There is no firewood available within the campground, but there are numerous areas nearby where you can gather firewood. There is no water here either; you have to haul in your own, so make sure you bring enough water to drink and douse your fire. Firewood and a water tap are available at Ray's General Store, 7 miles away in the sleepy little town of Tajique. The store is well stocked with groceries and sells gasoline; it also carries portable propane bottles and picnic supplies but no camping gear. The family who runs the store is nice, and the prices are reasonable.

## 28 Fourth of July Campground

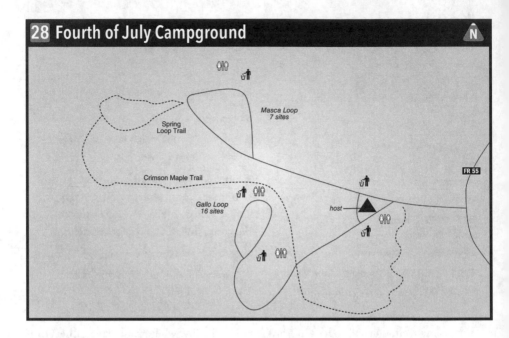

## :: Getting There

From NM 337 at the town of Tajique, turn at the campground sign, and follow FR 55 for 7 miles to the campground.

**GPS COORDINATES**   N34° 47.566'   W106° 22.984'

# 29

# Tajique Campground

*Tiny Tajique Creek gives this campground a magical ambience.*

**A** **small, pretty** campground awaits you just a few miles southwest of the tiny hamlet of Tajique (pronounced: tuh-hee-key). Tajique Campground has only five sites but is a comfortable campground nestled right off Forest Service Road 55. During the spring snowmelt, tiny Tajique Creek flows freely. There is no fishing, but it gives the campground a magical ambience. In May, the creek will dry up until the New Mexico monsoon season begins in July.

Enveloped in a forest of ponderosa pines, red cedars, piñons, alligator junipers, and Gambel oaks, the entire campground is shady. Outside of traffic passing on FR 55, the camp remains relatively quiet. Tajique is for tents, not RVs, and because of the parking configuration, the parking lot is too small for RVs. The only drawback is the Trigo Fire did extensive damage around this campground, but fortunately it left the campground itself intact. Flash flooding is a serious concern because of the massive Trigo burn scar.

Three of the five campsites are situated around the parking area, and two more are tucked back in the woods. Four sites have picnic tables and fire grates. The site against the fence is not very appealing (it will catch a fair amount of dust from the road), but the other four sites sit back from the road. The grassy streambed provides many good spots for setting up your tent.

There is a beautiful site across the stream, an easy 50-foot walk from the end of the loop. It sits apart from the other campsites and might be considered a "honeymoon suite." The other remote site is a 100-foot walk east of the vault toilet. This site has a rock fire ring but no picnic table. All of the sites are a decent size, and there is adequate privacy. There are a few short trails around the campground. With plenty of room to play, kids enjoy it here. The area is too small for bicycling, but kids can bike the trails.

There is no water, so bring an adequate supply of water to drink and douse your campfire. The vault toilet is clean and in good condition. Trash bins are bear-proof. There is no host, but the Forest Service patrols this area with some regularity, as does the Torrance County Sheriff's Department.

The campground has been picked clean of firewood, but you can gather adequate firewood along FR 55. In the town of Tajique, Ray's General Store is well stocked for groceries and also sells gasoline and picnic supplies but no camping gear. Prices are reasonable.

Because of the stream, beware of black bears, mountain lions, bobcats, raccoons, and coyotes. Needless to say, be sure to lock up all food items at night. Diamondback and prairie rattlesnakes inhabit the forests, so keep a close eye on children and pets.

## :: Ratings

BEAUTY: ★ ★ ★ ★
PRIVACY: ★ ★ ★ ★
SPACIOUSNESS: ★ ★ ★ ★
QUIET: ★ ★ ★
SECURITY: ★ ★ ★
CLEANLINESS: ★ ★ ★ ★ ★

## :: Key Information

**ADDRESS:** Cibola National Forest, Mountainair Ranger District, P.O. Box 69, Mountainair, NM 87036

**OPERATED BY:** U.S. Department of Agriculture

**CONTACT:** 505-847-2990; www.fs.usda.gov/cibola

**OPEN:** Year-round

**SITES:** 5

**SITE AMENITIES:** Fire ring, 4 with tables

**ASSIGNMENT:** First come, first served

**REGISTRATION:** Self-registration on-site

**FACILITIES:** Vault toilet; bring water.

**PARKING:** In parking area (max 5 vehicles)

**FEE:** None

**ELEVATION:** 7,048 feet

**RESTRICTIONS**

■ **Pets:** On 6-foot leash; take precautionary measures against predators.

■ **Fires:** In fire rings only; charcoal grills permitted; check with Forest Service office and postings on the camp bulletin board for restrictions.

■ **Alcohol:** No restrictions

■ **Other:** 14-day stay limit

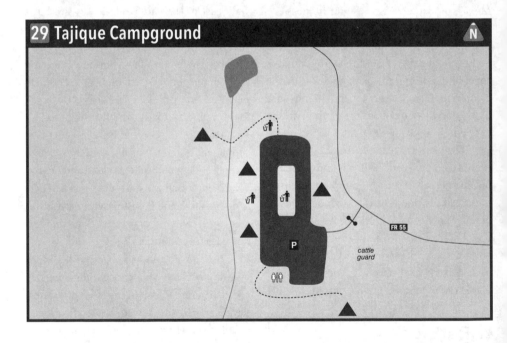

## :: Getting There

From NM 337 at Tajique, turn west onto FR 55 at the Fourth of July Campground sign. Drive 3 miles and turn left into the campground.

**GPS COORDINATES** N34° 45.954'  W106° 19.668'

# 30

# Caballo Lake State Park

*Riverside campsites are shaded by Russian olive, cottonwood, and salt cedar trees.*

**When people** think of lake camping in New Mexico, Elephant Butte Lake is the first place mentioned. But Elephant Butte is crowded, overdeveloped, and party central. A quieter choice is lovely Caballo Lake State Park, just 16 miles south of Elephant Butte. Caballo is New Mexico's third-largest state park and much more serene. Caballo campgrounds fill rapidly on the holidays, but tent campers always seem to find a space.

Caballo Lake was formed by an earth-filled dam that is 96 feet high and 4,558 feet long. Although Caballo Lake is shallow, with an average depth of 25 feet, the water surface area covers 11,500 acres and measures 18 miles long when at capacity. Depending on drought conditions, spillway gates are closed to preserve the precious water. During summer, the floodgates open to provide the fertile Mesilla (pronounced muh-see-uh) Valley, a few miles to the south, much-needed irrigation. This is where the delicious New Mexico green and red chiles are grown, along with many other crops. The Mesilla Valley is lush and green, a lovely oasis in the south-central New Mexico desert.

The Caballo Lake staff manages the crowds here well. The Sierra County Sheriff's Department and the New Mexico State Police patrol the campgrounds regularly. The U.S. Coast Guard Auxiliary has staff stationed here, and state park officers patrol the lake constantly. Pick up a boater's safety brochure because New Mexico boating laws have changed recently and are strictly enforced. This beautiful desert lake is a boater's paradise and is popular for fishing, water skiing, windsurfing, canoeing, kayaking, and inflatables.

Tent camping is provided at numerous areas. Some of the low-lying areas near the lake can flood, and the state park management will post signs prohibiting areas that are vulnerable. Many areas are considered primitive and permit dispersed tent camping. For tent campers, the best sites are found at Riverside Campground, on the south end of the dam. This is tent camping at its finest. From the entrance of this campground to the loop at the far end is exactly 1 mile. All of the best tent spots are located between the road and the Rio Grande. The riverside campsites are shady, with a mix of Russian olive, cottonwood, and salt cedar trees. The ground is level and sandy, with sparse wild grasses. You can pitch your tent right under the trees. The Youth Conservation Corps worked hard to install dozens of new shelters throughout

## :: Ratings

BEAUTY: ★ ★ ★ ★
PRIVACY: ★ ★ ★
SPACIOUSNESS: ★ ★ ★
QUIET: ★ ★ ★ ★
SECURITY: ★ ★ ★ ★ ★
CLEANLINESS: ★ ★ ★ ★ ★

## :: Key Information

**ADDRESS:** Caballo Lake State Park, US 187, Caballo, NM 87931

**OPERATED BY:** New Mexico State Parks

**CONTACT:** 575-743-3942; www.emnrd.state.nm.us/SPD /caballolakestatepark.html

**OPEN:** Year-round

**SITES:** 170

**SITE AMENITIES:** Parking space, picnic table, platform grill

**ASSIGNMENT:** First come, first served or reserve at **reserveamerica.com** or 877-664-7787.

**REGISTRATION:** At visitor center or self-registration on-site

**FACILITIES:** Visitor center

**PARKING:** At each site

**FEE:** $8 primitive, $10 nonelectric, $14 with electric or sewage hookup, $18 with electric and sewage hookups; $5 day-use fee per vehicle

**ELEVATION:** *Riverside* 4,172 feet; *Lake Office* 4,259 feet

**RESTRICTIONS**
■ **Pets:** On 10-foot leash; take precautionary measures against predators

■ **Fires:** No ground fires permitted; charcoal grills permitted

■ **Alcohol:** At campsites only; zero tolerance while boating

■ **Other:** Quiet hours 10 p.m.–8 a.m.; 21-day stay limit

the entire campground. Primitive camping is permitted here, and many sites are available without a picnic table or fire grate, but ground fires are not permitted. There is one comfort station equipped with flush toilets, sinks, and showers. One water spigot is located in front of the comfort station; 50 feet to the north is a modern playground.

Past the visitor center in the lakeside area are five camping areas for RVs separated from the tent areas. Two primitive camping areas are available for tent campers. Percha Flats Campground is located on the southwest corner of the lake below the dam. If the ground is dry, it makes for ideal beach camping. There is a large area for dispersed camping, but there are no picnic tables, fire rings, toilets, or shade. RVs are across the road and have a full hookup and water at each site. North of the boat dock, Upper Flats Beach Campground provides dispersed primitive camping with a few picnic tables and fire grates but little shade. Three portable outhouses are in this area.

You'll find an incredible cactus garden at the visitor center. The wide variety of cacti bloom in April and May. More than 200 species of birds and waterfowl thrive here, including the sandhill crane. Bald and golden eagles roost here seasonally, following other waterfowl migrations. Turkey vultures are a common sight, scavenging for fish. The park is also home to coyotes, several squirrel species, rabbits, foxes, raccoons, mule deer, black bears, rattlesnakes, lizards, frogs, and turtles. Bobcats and mountain lions have been spotted in the Caballo Mountains but usually shy away from the park.

In summer, you can expect temperatures in the 100°F range, but it cools down to the 70s at night. Thunderstorms are rare until July, when the monsoon season is welcomed here in the Chihuahuan Desert. The sunsets are incredible; the pink and orange horizon sets the Caballo Mountains in fiery red nearly every evening. The night skies are wide open, so it's a stargazer's paradise; bring your telescope.

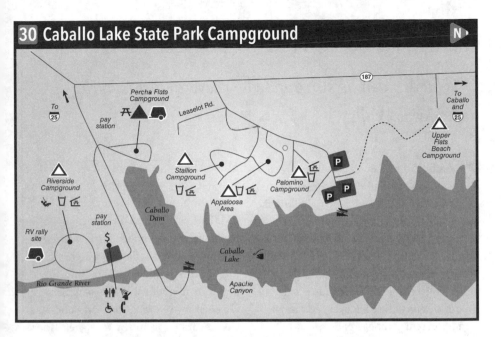

## 30 Caballo Lake State Park Campground

## :: Getting There

From Truth or Consequences, take I-25 south 16 miles to Exit 59 and follow the signs. There are two entrances: the north entrance leads to the visitor center and lakeside campgrounds, and the south entrance leads to the dam road and Riverside Campground.

**GPS COORDINATES   Lakeside Visitor Center   N32° 53.764'   W107° 18.547'**

# 31

# Percha Dam State Park

*This hidden gem is surrounded by several farms in the lush Mesilla Valley.*

**P**ercha Dam State Park features a beautiful, quiet, small campground located just a scant 3 miles south of Caballo Lake State Park. It is a hidden gem, surrounded by several farms in the lush Mesilla Valley. Named for Percha Creek, which flows into the Rio Grande, this serene park provides an ideal place to kick back and relax to the sound of water cascading over the dam. It's a wonderful tent camper's park.

Tent camping is dispersed, and there are no marked or numbered sites. Just set up the tent where you wish and enjoy the lush grass and shade of the cottonwood, river willow, Russian olive, ash, and salt cedar trees. Several sites along the Rio Grande provide excellent shade, grass, a few picnic tables, and fire rings. Many dispersed tent sites lie under tall cottonwood trees in the grass meadow between the roads. These sites are on a slight downslope. Water runoff flows into a small canal dividing the meadow area in half. This meadow is ideal for tents, but there is little to no privacy between sites. A group shelter houses

a dozen picnic tables and a fireplace. It provides an excellent escape from afternoon summer rains.

The park offers an immaculate comfort station equipped with flush toilets, sinks, and showers. Several water spigots are located throughout the park, and the state performs frequent water tests. The RV area (all sites have electric and water hookups) is well separated from the tent sites. There is no firewood here; you must bring your own. Plenty of parking is available.

Security is excellent. A campground host is on-site, and the area is patrolled by New Mexico State Parks, New Mexico State Police, Sierra County Sheriff's Department, and New Mexico game wardens. Have your fishing license available at all times.

If you feel like a little exercise, check out the short 0.5-mile hiking trail within the park. Percha Dam State Park is known as a prime bird-watcher's paradise. You will see various species of ducks, geese, herons, cranes, and swans. Sightings of golden and bald eagles, a variety of hawks, and falcons are also common here. The elusive peregrine falcon makes its aerie in the nearby Caballo Mountains. You may spot occasional deer, coyotes, raccoons, red foxes, rabbits, and squirrels throughout the area.

Swimming is not recommended here because of the swift current of the Rio Grande, but canoeing, rafting, and kayaking are excellent. All occupants in the watercraft

## :: Ratings

BEAUTY: ★ ★ ★ ★
PRIVACY: ★ ★ ★
SPACIOUSNESS: ★ ★ ★ ★
QUIET: ★ ★ ★ ★
SECURITY: ★ ★ ★ ★ ★
CLEANLINESS: ★ ★ ★ ★ ★

## :: Key Information

| | |
|---|---|
| **ADDRESS:** US 187, Caballo, NM 87931 | **FACILITIES:** Restrooms, showers, vault toilets, visitor center |
| **OPERATED BY:** New Mexico State Parks | **PARKING:** At each site |
| **CONTACT:** 575-743-3942; www.emnrd.state.nm.us/SPD /perchadamstatepark.html | **FEE:** $8 primitive, $10 nonelectric, $14 with electric or sewage hookup, $18 with electric and sewage hookups; $5 day-use fee per vehicle |
| **OPEN:** Year-round | |
| **SITES:** 50 | **ELEVATION:** 4,149 feet |
| **SITE AMENITIES:** Parking space, picnic table, fire ring | **RESTRICTIONS** |
| **ASSIGNMENT:** First come, first served or reserve at **reserveamerica.com** or 877-664-7787. | ■ **Pets:** On 10-foot leash |
| | ■ **Fires:** No ground fires; charcoal grills permitted |
| **REGISTRATION:** Self-registration on-site without a reservation; with reservation, follow instructions on website and print receipt of reservation for check-in. | ■ **Alcohol:** At campsites only |
| | ■ **Other:** Quiet hours 10 p.m.–8 a.m.; 14-day stay limit |

must wear a personal flotation device—no exceptions. Fishing in the small pond is fair for bass, catfish, and occasional walleye. No swimming is permitted in the nearby irrigation canals because of possible pesticide contamination in the water. The state of New Mexico has made some significant improvements here, including a modern playground at the park's south end.

Temperatures often exceed 100°F in summer, but with shade trees, summer breezes, and low humidity, it is still pleasant. Folks drive to Caballo Lake to swim or canoe for the day to escape the heat. Nights cool off into the 70s in the summer, with gentle breezes. Occasional thunderstorms begin in July and cool things off. I love walking in the warm summer rain.

The small town of Hatch, New Mexico, is 18 miles south, off I-25. It's an excellent place for supplies. The town is the main entry point of the Mesilla Valley, and the produce here is incredible. In the fall, apples, peaches, and apricots are available. Also try the pistachio and almond nuts grown here and sold all year. You will be amazed at the variety of New Mexico chile products to sample, including green chile chocolate candy!

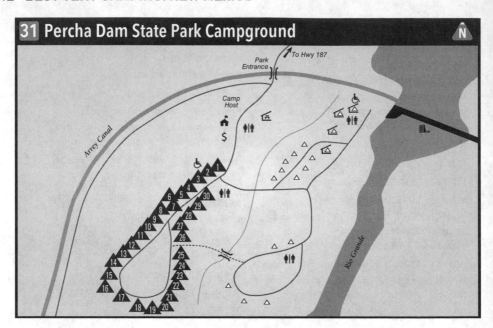

## :: Getting There

Take I-25 to Exit 59. Follow NM 187 south 2 miles, turn left at the Percha Dam sign, and follow the road 1 mile to the campground.

**GPS COORDINATES**   N32° 52.133'   W107° 18.356'

# 32

# Aguirre Springs Recreation Area

*Aguirre Springs offers a unique Chihuahuan Desert camping experience.*

**P**erched high in the foothills beneath the towering cathedral spires of the Organ Mountains, beautiful Aguirre Springs Recreation Area is a must for those seeking a Chihuahuan Desert camping experience. This is the only high-country campground in the area, and it's conveniently located 17 miles east of Las Cruces.

Aguirre Springs Campground gets busy on weekends. Campsites serve as picnic sites for Las Cruces residents. The campground attracts a few RVs but is designed mainly for tent campers. It's divided into two loops: the main loop and the east loop. All sites accommodate tents, but some sites in the main loop are not level. There is no grass, and the ground can be rocky in spots. The most level sites are in the east loop, and there is more privacy there away from the picnic crowds. Most sites have privacy due to trees and native desert bushes. Many new steel shelters have been added to provide shade in sites where trees are not present. Three modern vault toilets are spaced throughout

## :: Ratings

> BEAUTY: ★ ★ ★ ★
> PRIVACY: ★ ★ ★
> SPACIOUSNESS: ★ ★ ★
> QUIET: ★ ★ ★ ★
> SECURITY: ★ ★ ★ ★
> CLEANLINESS: ★ ★ ★ ★ ★

camp. Gathering firewood is prohibited here, but firewood is sold at the camp host's residence, where the water supply is also located, to the right before you enter the campground.

Aguirre Springs is scenic, and the early-morning sunlight catches the Organ Mountains best for pictures. White Sands Missile Range and the Tularosa Valley provide majestic views to the north and east. Yucca blooms appear in April through mid-June, when native cacti and succulent plants flower at the same time. Piñon and juniper trees dot the rugged hillsides, adding a lovely hue of green to the gray and tan of the Organ Mountains. Alligator juniper, gray oak, and mountain mahogany provide shade. Dwarf mesquite trees are native here.

Mule deer, oryx, and pronghorn antelope are common. Visits by mountain lions have become more frequent, so beware. Rattlesnakes are also common here, so brush up on how to avoid them. Keep your tents zipped tightly shut at all times. Several species of scorpions and centipedes are also residents you'll want to avoid.

Two hiking trails are featured in the Aguirre Springs Recreation Area: 6-mile Baylor Pass Trail takes you to the other side of the Organ Mountains, and 4-mile Pine Tree Trail takes you into a ponderosa pine and spruce forest. Both trails offer great views of the Tularosa Basin. White Sands National

## :: Key Information

| | |
|---|---|
| **ADDRESS:** Las Cruces District Office, 1800 Marquess St., Las Cruces, NM 88005-3370 | **FACILITIES:** Restrooms |
| | **PARKING:** At each site |
| **OPERATED BY:** Bureau of Land Management | **FEE:** $7, $50 group site; $5 day-use fee |
| | **ELEVATION:** 5,639 feet |
| **CONTACT:** 575-525-4300; **blm.gov** | **RESTRICTIONS** |
| **OPEN:** Year-round; April–Oct., entrance gate open 8 a.m.–8 p.m.; Oct.–April, 8 a.m.–6 p.m. | ■ **Pets:** On 6-foot leash; take precautionary measures against predators. |
| **SITES:** 57 | ■ **Fires:** In fire rings only; charcoal grills permitted; check with campground host, BLM office, and postings on the camp bulletin board for restrictions. |
| **SITE AMENITIES:** Parking space, trashcan, picnic table, fire ring; some with metal shelters and pedestal grills | |
| **ASSIGNMENT:** First come, first served. | ■ **Alcohol:** At campsites only |
| **REGISTRATION:** Self-registration on-site | ■ **Other:** Quiet hours 10 p.m.–8 a.m.; 14-day stay limit |

Monument is 34 miles north on US 70 and is a must-see. It is a playground of pure white gypsum sand and an enjoyable day trip.

Summers here can be quite hot, exceeding 100°F. The ideal camping season is spring because of the blooming yucca and cacti. Fall is pleasant but can be quite windy. Expect spring and fall daytime temperatures in the 70°F range, while nights drop into the 50s.

Winter can be quite cold here, dropping as low as 20°F at night, and snow is possible anytime from November through March. Daytime temperatures in winter are 40°F–60°F. The Las Cruces Bureau of Land Management, Dona Ana County Sheriff's Department, and the New Mexico State Police patrol frequently, and a camp host is present within 0.5 mile of the main campground.

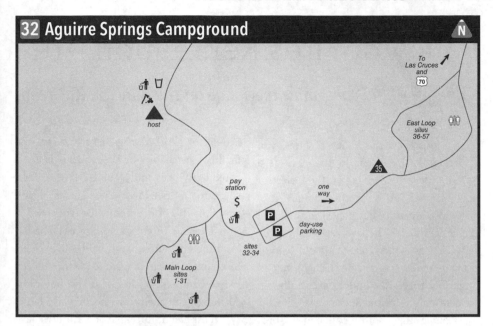

## :: Getting There

From Las Cruces, travel 17 miles east on US 70. The turnoff, marked by a large sign, is on the south side of the highway. At mile 4, the road becomes a one-way loop; travel another 2 miles to the campground. The road is paved to the campground, but the drive is slow due to the many tight turns you will encounter.

**GPS COORDINATES**  N32° 22.250'  W106° 33.657'

# 33

# Valley of Fires Recreation Area

*A one-of-a-kind camping experience on the Billy the Kid Trail.*

**A**s you view the Valley of Fires, you might ask, "What in the heck is a Hawaiian lava field doing in the desert of New Mexico?" It is another unique joke that Mother Nature has played in the Land of Enchantment. The lava is thought to be between 2,000 and 5,000 years old (geologists are unable to agree on the age), but all agree that this is the youngest lava flow in the continental United States.

Containing both pahoehoe (pronounced puh-hoy-hoy) and a'a' (pronounced ah ah) lava common to the Hawaiian Islands, this incredible landscape is both eerie and beautiful. The lava flow extends for 44 miles, is 2–5 miles wide along the Tularosa Valley, and has a surface area of 127 square miles. The lava is believed to be 165 feet thick at its deepest point. Wildflowers, yucca, cholla, prickly pear, and many shrub species common to the Chihuahuan Desert thrive here, their beautiful green hue contrasting against the brash black lava.

Valley of Fires Campground is a one-of-a-kind camping experience. The campground was originally a New Mexico State Park established in 1966. Years later, the

Bureau of Land Management obtained the facility. The majority of the acreage is dedicated to RV sites, and all have electric power, so there's no need to use generators. A sign prohibits RVs from entering the tent area.

The six-site tent-camping area is shaded by juniper, piñon, and wild olive trees. Sites are separated from one another by trees, scrub oak bushes, and lava boulders. Although the sites aren't particularly large, two tents can fit into each one. All sites have a gravel tent box, a nice grassy area, and a picnic table covered by a steel shade shelter. Across the road is a modern vault toilet.

Past the tent area is a large day-use area, with a group shelter, picnic tables, pedestal grills, and a sand volleyball pit. Hilltop Vista Overlook is a great place to catch a glimpse of the massive lava field to the north, east, and west, as well as the entire campground.

The main restroom is typical of New Mexico State Park comfort stations—roomy and sparkling clean with flush toilets, sinks, and warm-water showers. Four water spigots are available to tent campers, and each RV site has its own water spigot. The water here is Carrizozo city water.

The 0.75-mile hiking trail leads into the heart of the lava flow, and interpretive signs identify plants, flowers, and interesting facts along the trail. Trail maps are free at the Valley of Fires Visitor Center, which also has books, T-shirts, gifts, and information about public lands in New Mexico.

The desert sometimes exceeds 100°F in summer. Fall, winter, and spring are

## :: Ratings

BEAUTY: ★ ★ ★
PRIVACY: ★ ★ ★ ★
SPACIOUSNESS: ★ ★ ★
QUIET: ★ ★ ★ ★ ★
SECURITY: ★ ★ ★ ★ ★
CLEANLINESS: ★ ★ ★ ★ ★

## :: Key Information

**ADDRESS:** P.O. Box 871, Carrizozo, NM 88301

**OPERATED BY:** Bureau of Land Management

**CONTACT:** 575-648-2242; **blm.gov**

**OPEN:** Year-round

**SITES:** 14 RV sites; 6 tent sites

**SITE AMENITIES:** Parking space, picnic table, fire ring, tent box, shelter

**ASSIGNMENT:** First come, first served

**REGISTRATION:** Self-registration on-site

**FACILITIES:** Restrooms, showers, vault toilets, visitor center

**PARKING:** At each site

**FEE:** $10 per family per day; $3 per adult (16 and older) per day; children 15 and under free

**ELEVATION:** 5,710 feet

**RESTRICTIONS**

■ **Pets:** On 6-foot leash; not allowed on nature trails; this is black bear country and also home to mountain lions, bobcats, and coyotes, so monitor pets closely.

■ **Fires:** In fire rings only; charcoal grills permitted; check with campground host, Forest Service office, and postings on the camp bulletin board for restrictions.

■ **Alcohol:** At campsites only

■ **Other:** Quiet hours 10 p.m.–8 a.m.; 14-day stay limit

wonderful times to visit. A campground host is assigned here year-round. No firewood is available, so bring your own or buy firewood in nearby Carrizozo. While in Carrizozo, try a bottle of the delicious cherry cider and taste the pecans, almonds, pistachios, peaches, cherries, apricots, and apples grown in nearby orchards.

### Nearby Attraction

**GHOST TOWN OF WHITE OAKS, NM:**

**Hot on the Trail of Billy the Kid**

In 1878, gold was discovered outside White Oaks, and very quickly the town became incredibly wealthy and wild. Prospering from several highly profitable gold mines located at nearby Baxter Mountain to the west and Lone Mountain to the north, the prospectors came to White Oaks. The town's population reached its peak at around 2,500 by 1895.

White Oaks became one of Billy the Kid's favorite haunts. "With all of its brothels and casinos, Billy the Kid thought of White Oaks as a resort," stated historian Drew Gomber. Things were fine with Billy coming into town and enjoying the ambience, until he and his gang became suspects for stealing horses in White Oaks. Several attempts were made to capture them, but none succeeded.

At the height of the Lincoln County war, on April 28th, 1881, Billy escaped jail in the nearby town of Lincoln. During the escape, he shot and killed Deputy Sheriff James W. Bell, and a few minutes later, he assassinated Sheriff Robert Ollinger. James Bell was buried in the Cedarvale Cemetery in White Oaks. Cedarvale Cemetery also holds the bodies of 11 men killed in a mining accident, along with other noted military veterans and townspeople.

After the Lincoln County War, Susan McSween Barber, widow of Alexander McSween, one of the leaders of the Regulators (Billy's faction in the war), became the only individual to profit from the war. She acquired an enormous amount of land after the war ended and maintained 3,000–5,000 head of cattle on her nearby ranch. She was known as the "Cattle Queen" of New Mexico. In 1902 she sold her holdings and moved to White Oaks, retiring as a very wealthy woman. She died there on January 3, 1931, and is also buried in the Cedarvale Cemetery.

By the time of her death, the gold mines had played out, and the town was abandoned except for a few hearty souls. Today, the town's population is 22. White Oaks remains a popular place to visit, and there are two magnificent homes, built around the time that Billy was alive. The Hoyle House and the Gumm House can be photographed from the road. They are both occupied; please respect the owners' privacy. Also check out the four-room schoolhouse that is now a museum, and some old crumbling adobe structures and several dilapidated houses that make excellent subjects for shutterbugs.

The No Scum Allowed Saloon serves food as well as adult beverages on weekends, and one small store sells snacks, sodas, and antiques. White Oaks artist Bob Reynierson is an impressionist painter, sculptor, and sometimes gold miner who owns a studio, and Ivy Heymann's studio features pottery. At the Miners Home and Toolshed Museum you can view authentic furnishings and real mining tools. For more information about White Oaks, visit **whiteoaks.com.**

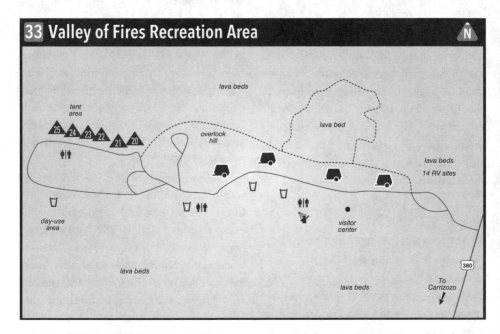

## :: Getting There

From Carrizozo, drive northwest on US 54 for 3.8 miles to the turnoff for NM 349, known as the White Oaks Highway. Continue up White Oaks Highway for 8.2 miles to the ghost town. Valley of Fires National Recreation Area is 4 miles west of Carrizozo, south off US 380.

**GPS COORDINATES**   N33° 41.052'   W105° 55.228'

# Oak Grove Campground

*Enjoy the serenity of the wind in the pines at Oak Grove.*

**A**way from the madding crowds of Ruidoso, quiet Oak Grove Campground awaits just east of Alto, New Mexico. This is the White Mountain Wilderness Area, within the Sacramento Mountain Range. Here it is peaceful and wild. You can enjoy the serenity of the wind in the pines and a large meadow filled with wild iris and bright green native grasses dancing in the cool mountain breezes. I awoke at 4 a.m. to the sound of a pack of coyotes singing.

Forest fire damage seen to the northwest of the camp is just one of many scars upon the mountains of Southern New Mexico. Despite the fire damage, this campground is still lovely. Sierra Blanca Peak is 3 miles from Oak Grove as the crow flies.

Shaded by piñon, juniper, Gambel oak, and spruce trees, Oak Grove features 30 sites that are exceptionally well designed for tents. RVs longer than 18 feet are discouraged from the campground. The campground is private, with several campsites hidden among the rocks. There is a host's site, but it may not be occupied. Most sites have a gravel area for the fire pit and picnic table. All sites are level and have plenty of shade. There are three modern vault toilets and plenty of firewood, but no water. The only downside of Oak Grove is its lack of security. There may be no host, and I never saw any Forest Service patrols.

Oak Grove is incredible in the fall—the oak leaves turn a fiery orange. Several herds of wild horses are native to the Sacramento Mountains. The horses often migrate to this meadow to graze. Elk are common, and their mating calls can be heard during the fall rut. Bears, mountain lions, and bobcats also frequent Oak Grove, so keep a clean camp.

A beautiful drive to the Mescalero Apache Tribe's Ski Apache resort down NM 532 is a must. The road has several hairpin turns and is not for the faint of heart, but the views are incredible—this is the New Mexico people want to see. Elk and deer are common along the drive, so be careful.

The elevation dramatically increases from 8,400 feet at the campground to 10,066 feet at the road's summit. The road then descends to the ski basin at 9,700 feet. The summit house is at 11,280 feet, and the highest point of Sierra Blanca Peak is 11,549 feet. This is an incredible hiking opportunity; do not forget your camera.

Eagle Lake Campground, south of NM 532, is run by the Mescalero Apache Tribe. The camp offers fishing ponds and rustic camping with 20 sites. Nearby Skyline Campground with 17 campsites and the Monjeau Overlook Picnic Grounds on Forest Service Road 117 can be accessed by high-clearance vehicles only.

## :: Ratings

BEAUTY: ★ ★ ★ ★ ★
PRIVACY: ★ ★ ★ ★ ★
SPACIOUSNESS: ★ ★ ★ ★ ★
QUIET: ★ ★ ★ ★ ★
SECURITY: ★
CLEANLINESS: ★ ★ ★ ★ ★

## :: Key Information

**ADDRESS:** Lincoln National Forest, Smokey Bear Ranger District, 901 Mechem, Ruidoso, NM 88345

**OPERATED BY:** U.S. Department of Agriculture

**CONTACT:** 575-257-4095; **www.fs.usda.gov/lincoln**

**OPEN:** May 15–Sept. 30

**SITES:** 30, 1 group site (accommodates 20–50 people)

**SITE AMENITIES:** Parking space, picnic table, fire ring

**ASSIGNMENT:** First come, first served

**REGISTRATION:** Self-registration on-site

**FACILITIES:** Vault toilets; bring water.

**PARKING:** At each site

**FEE:** $6, plus $6 per night for each additional vehicle (2 vehicles max)

**ELEVATION:** 8,496 feet

**RESTRICTIONS**

■ **Pets:** On leash; take precautionary measures against predators

■ **Fires:** In fire rings only; charcoal grills permitted; check with campground host, Forest Service office, and postings on the camp bulletin board for restrictions.

■ **Alcohol:** At campsites only

■ **Other:** Quiet hours 10 p.m.–8 a.m.; 14-day stay limit

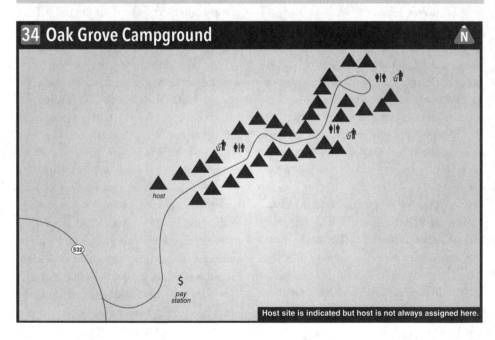

**34** Oak Grove Campground

host

532

$
pay
station

Host site is indicated but host is not always assigned here.

## :: Getting There

Follow NM 48 north out of Ruidoso for 4 miles; turn left (west) on NM 532 and go 5 miles to Oak Grove.

**GPS COORDINATES** N33° 23.562'  W105° 44.983'

# 35

# Silver Lake Campground

*Sleep under a canopy of ponderosa pine, oak, juniper, blue spruce, fir, and aspen trees.*

**F**or those who love primitive camping in a lovely setting, Silver Lake Campground on the Mescalero Apache Reservation is waiting for you. The privilege of camping on Native American land is always a thrill. It is like stepping back in time. There is no cellular service or Internet access here. The only link to the outside world is a pay telephone.

The Mescalero Apache Tribe has three subtribes: the Mescalero, the Chiricahua, and the Lipan. Mescalero tribal lands encompass 720 square miles of beautiful mountain wilderness. The Mescalero business enterprises include the Inn of the Mountain Gods Resort & Casino, the Apache Nugget Casino, and the Ski Apache resort. About 4,000 tribal members live on Mescalero land.

The friendly and helpful staff openly welcome campers. The campground office is an A-frame cabin with a small store selling basic groceries, including ice and firewood. There is no firewood to gather within the camp. The camp has no paved or gravel roads but is pleasant, and the surrounding mountains are beautiful. There are many shady areas for tent campers under the canopy of ponderosa pine, oak, juniper, blue spruce, fir, and aspen trees. About 100 areas exist to pitch a tent, and it's easy to find a remote site that is level. RVs are not permitted in the tent area, and no tents are allowed in the RV area. All RV sites have electrical hookups, and generators are not permitted.

There is a small playground in the meadow between the RV area and the tent area. Portable toilets are distributed throughout the camp, and tent campers have their own bathhouse complete with sinks, flush toilets, and warm-water showers. Fresh water spigots are located at the entrance of the camp, and the water should be filtered. Each camper gets a color map of the grounds and a short list of practical campground rules. The campground is administered similar to a private campground and is kept clean. Mescalero police and Federal Conservation officers have jurisdiction here and ensure safety.

Fishing is good here. The 7-acre lake is stocked every two weeks with rainbow trout raised at the nearby fish hatchery, which is also operated by the tribe. Because this is a reservation lake, New Mexico fishing licenses are not required, and a fishing permit is $10, with a limit of five trout per permit.

## :: Ratings

BEAUTY: ★ ★ ★ ★ ★
PRIVACY: ★ ★ ★ ★ ★
SPACIOUSNESS: ★ ★ ★ ★ ★
QUIET: ★ ★ ★ ★ ★
SECURITY: ★ ★ ★ ★ ★
CLEANLINESS: ★ ★ ★ ★ ★

## :: Key Information

**ADDRESS:** Mescalero Apache Reservation, 868 NM 244, Mescalero, NM 88340

**OPERATED BY:** Mescalero Apache Reservation

**CONTACT:** 575-464-2244

**OPEN:** First week of April–last week of Sept.

**SITES:** 150 acres, dispersed

**SITE AMENITIES:** Picnic table, fire ring

**ASSIGNMENT:** First come, first served

**REGISTRATION:** At office prior to entry

**FACILITIES:** Restrooms, showers

**PARKING:** Ample spaces

**FEE:** RV: $15 per night for first 2 people per vehicle and 50 cents each additional person; tent: $12 per night for first 2 people per vehicle and 50 cents each additional person

**ELEVATION:** 7,640 feet

**RESTRICTIONS**

■ **Pets:** On 6-foot leash; take precautionary measures against predators.

■ **Fires:** In fire rings only; charcoal grills permitted

■ **Alcohol:** May not be permitted; ask the front office before indulging.

■ **Other:** Quiet hours 11 p.m.–8 a.m.

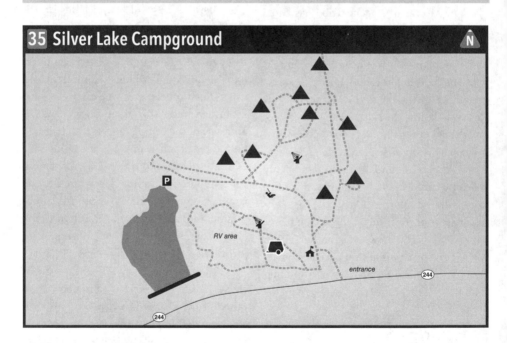

**35 Silver Lake Campground**

RV area

entrance

244

244

## :: Getting There

From Cloudcroft, take NM 82 west 1 mile, and turn north on NM 244 for 8 miles. The campground is on the left side of road.

**GPS COORDINATES**   N33° 1.082'   W105° 37.745'

# 36

# Pines Campground

*Pines is a delightful tent-camper's haven.*

**P**ines Campground is my number one pick of all the campgrounds in Lincoln National Forest. This is a delightful tent camper's haven, just 1.25 miles north of the town of Cloudcroft. Cloudcroft is a lively town of more than 700 residents. It offers two golf courses, a miniature golf course, and two astronomical observatories nearby. The Mexican Trestle, an old railroad trestle built across a steep canyon, is a popular attraction. Wi-Fi is available at the Cloudcroft Chamber of Commerce building. Mountaintop Mercantile is a full-service grocery store with camping supplies. Cloudcroft has several gasoline stations, a couple of restaurants, and an ice-cream shop and candy store for those with a sweet tooth.

Situated in a forest of mature ponderosa pines and a few spruce, fir, and Gambel oak trees, Pines Campground is quite shady. All sites are on the outside of the loop, which means plenty of space between sites for privacy. Each site comes equipped with a new-style fire ring and picnic table. The double and triple sites are equipped with pedestal grills. The parking pads are only large enough to accommodate 16-foot trailers, and there will be a few pop-up campers. Most campsites are grassy. Three wheelchair-accessible vault toilets are spotless and conveniently spaced, with water spigots and varmint-proof trash bins. The water is Cloudcroft City water.

The campground is more than 8,600 feet in elevation, so be prepared for cool nights that occasionally dip into the 40°F range. The only drawback here is the road noise from NM 244, but the highway quiets down after dark, so you will have a peaceful evening by the campfire.

A camp host is assigned here, and the Forest Service and Otero County Sheriff's Department conduct frequent patrols. Plus, there is cellular service at the campground. Black bears can be common here, so you should stow all food-related items unless preparing meals or eating. You may hear coyotes and owls during the night. Blue jays are common, as are hummingbirds, so bring your feeders.

## :: Ratings

BEAUTY: ★ ★ ★ ★ ★
PRIVACY: ★ ★ ★ ★ ★
SPACIOUSNESS: ★ ★ ★ ★ ★
QUIET: ★ ★ ★
SECURITY: ★ ★ ★ ★ ★
CLEANLINESS: ★ ★ ★ ★ ★

## :: Key Information

**ADDRESS:** Lincoln National Forest, Sacramento Ranger District, 4 Lodge Rd., Cloudcroft, NM 88317

**OPERATED BY:** U.S. Department of Agriculture

**CONTACT:** 575-682-2551; **www.fs.usda.gov/lincoln**

**OPEN:** May 17–Sept. 3

**SITES:** 24

**SITE AMENITIES:** Parking space, picnic table, fire ring; some have pedestal grill.

**ASSIGNMENT:** First come, first served

**REGISTRATION:** Self-registration on-site

**FACILITIES:** Vault toilets

**PARKING:** At each site

**FEE:** $20 1-family unit, $25 2-family unit, $32 3-family unit, $38 4-family unit; $9 per night for each additional vehicle; showers available at Silver Campground for $5 per person

**ELEVATION:** 8,634 feet

**RESTRICTIONS**

■ **Pets:** On 6-foot leash; take precautionary measures against predators.

■ **Fires:** In fire rings only; charcoal grills permitted

■ **Alcohol:** At campsites only

■ **Other:** Quiet hours 10 p.m.–8 a.m.; 14-day stay limit

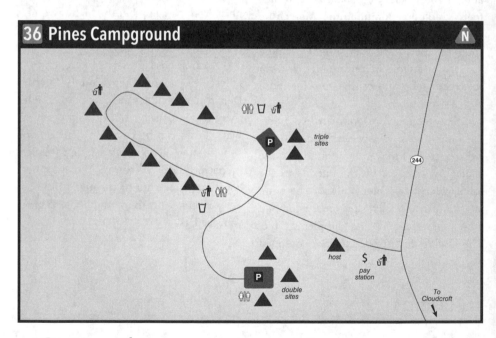

**36 Pines Campground**

## :: Getting There

From Cloudcroft, drive 1.25 miles north on NM 244. The campground turnoff is marked with a sign, to your left.

**GPS COORDINATES**   N32° 58.002'   W105° 44.109'

# 37

# Deerhead Campground

*This woodland paradise is very conducive to tent camping.*

**D**eerhead Campground was recently renovated, and they did a great job with the landscaping. It is just like camping in a woodland paradise and is very conducive to tent camping. Blue jays are common, as are hummingbirds, so bring your feeders.

After entering the campground, you will drive past the campground host's site and the pay station and bulletin board. The camp is well shaded with a healthy stand of ponderosa pine and fir trees. Turning left, you enter the shorter loop. Sites 1, 2, 4, 5, 6, and 8 are single sites; 7 is designated for disabled campers; and site 3 is a double site. Sites around this loop experience more traffic noise because of its close proximity to NM 130. Since the sites are closer together, there will be less privacy, but it would be a good area to camp close to friends or other family members.

From the entrance road, if you turn right, you will enter the longer loop. On this loop, there will be less traffic noise, as the loop is farther away from the highway. The sites are spaced much farther apart, affording more privacy. Elk are frequent visitors, as are black bears, so practice safe food storage.

While visiting the busy and quaint town of Cloudcroft, you will discover some fun attractions, including the Sunspot Observatory. The Mexican Trestle is an interesting look into the past, and the old railroad trestle has been restored. The Cloudcroft Chamber of Commerce provides Wi-Fi. Mountaintop Mercantile is a grocery store that carries camping gear. Cloudcroft also features two golf courses, a miniature golf course, several service stations, several restaurants (including a barbecue joint), and even a candy store and an ice cream shop.

This campground always has a host, and the Forest Service and Otero County Sheriff's Department frequently patrol the area. Since you are close to Cloudcroft, there is cellular service at the campground.

## :: Ratings

BEAUTY: ★ ★ ★ ★ ★
PRIVACY: ★ ★ ★ ★ ★
SPACIOUSNESS: ★ ★ ★ ★ ★
QUIET: ★ ★ ★
SECURITY: ★ ★ ★ ★ ★
CLEANLINESS: ★ ★ ★ ★ ★

## :: Key Information

**ADDRESS:** Lincoln National Forest, Sacramento Ranger District, 4 Lodge Rd., Cloudcroft, NM 88317

**OPERATED BY:** U.S. Department of Agriculture

**CONTACT:** 575-682-2551; www.fs.usda.gov/lincoln

**OPEN:** May 17–Sept. 3

**SITES:** 20

**SITE AMENITIES:** Picnic table, fire ring, pedestal grill, parking spur

**ASSIGNMENT:** First come, first served

**REGISTRATION:** Self-registration on-site

**FACILITIES:** Vault toilets, central garbage depository

**PARKING:** At each site

**FEE:** $18; $9 per night for each additional vehicle; showers available at Silver Campground for $5 per person

**ELEVATION:** 8,751 feet

**RESTRICTIONS**

■ **Pets:** On 6-foot leash; take precautionary measures against predators.

■ **Fires:** In fire rings only; charcoal grills permitted; check with campground host, Forest Service office, and postings on the camp bulletin board for restrictions.

■ **Alcohol:** At campsites only

■ **Other:** Quiet hours 10 p.m.–8 a.m.; 14-day stay limit

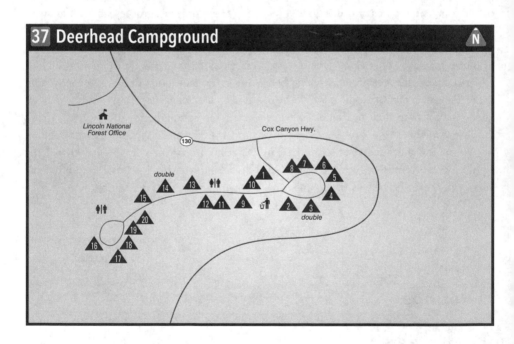

**37 Deerhead Campground**

## :: Getting There

From Cloudcroft, drive south on NM 130 for 1.2 miles to the campground sign.

**GPS COORDINATES**   N32° 56.622'   W105° 44.783'

# 38

# Sleepy Grass Campground

*Sleepy Grass Campground is located along a grassy valley cradled between mountains.*

**Sleepy Grass** Campground is much larger than Deerhead but every bit as beautiful. It is located along a grassy valley cradled between mountainsides and shaded by ponderosa pines, Douglas firs, and aspens. Blue jays are common, as well as hummingbirds, so bring your feeders.

Sleepy Grass has a large number of walk-in sites. Sites 3, 10, 12, and 19 are double sites; the rest are single sites. The camp is well shaded with a healthy stand of ponderosa pine and fir trees. Water spigots are located at the host site, near the vault toilets near site 4, near walk-in sites 8–12, and at the far end of the campground. Elk and mule deer are frequent visitors, as are black bears, so practice safe food storage and keep an eye on young children and pets.

The nearby town of Cloudcroft features some fun attractions, including the Sunspot Observatory. The Mexican Trestle is an interesting look into the past, and the old railroad trestle has been restored. The Cloudcroft Chamber of Commerce provides Wi-Fi. Mountaintop Mercantile is a grocery store that carries camping gear. Cloudcroft also features two golf courses, a miniature golf course, several service stations, several restaurants (including a barbecue joint), and even a candy store and an ice cream shop.

This campground always has a host, and the Forest Service and Otero County Sheriff's Department frequently patrol the area. Since you are close to Cloudcroft, there is cellular service at the campground.

## :: Ratings

BEAUTY: ★ ★ ★ ★ ★
PRIVACY: ★ ★ ★ ★ ★
SPACIOUSNESS: ★ ★ ★ ★ ★
QUIET: ★ ★ ★
SECURITY: ★ ★ ★ ★ ★
CLEANLINESS: ★ ★ ★ ★ ★

## :: Key Information

**ADDRESS:** Lincoln National Forest, Sacramento Ranger District, 4 Lodge Rd., Cloudcroft, NM 88317

**OPERATED BY:** U.S. Department of Agriculture

**CONTACT:** 575-682-2551; **www.fs.usda.gov/lincoln**

**OPEN:** May 17–Sept. 3

**SITES:** 21

**SITE AMENITIES:** Picnic table, fire ring, pedestal grill, parking spur

**ASSIGNMENT:** First come, first served

**REGISTRATION:** Self-registration on-site

**FACILITIES:** Vault toilets, central garbage depository

**PARKING:** At each site

**FEE:** $18 single, $23 double; $9 per night for each additional vehicle; showers available at Silver Campground for $5 per person

**ELEVATION:** 9,004 feet

**RESTRICTIONS**

■ **Pets:** On 6-foot leash; take precautionary measures against predators.

■ **Fires:** In fire rings only; charcoal grills permitted; check with campground host, Forest Service office, and postings on the camp bulletin board for restrictions.

■ **Alcohol:** At campsites only

■ **Other:** Quiet hours 10 p.m.–8 a.m.; 14-day stay limit

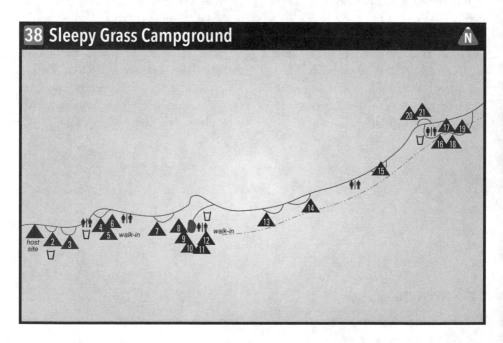

## :: Getting There

From Cloudcroft, drive 1.3 miles south on NM 130 to the campground sign.

**GPS COORDINATES**   N32° 56.939'   W105° 43.166'

# 39

# Sumner Lake State Park

*Don't miss this refreshing desert lake on the Trail of Billy the Kid.*

**The drive** to Sumner Lake State Park is delightful. As you travel US 84, you'll see hundreds of cattle grazing in the tall prairie grass. Once at the park, to reach the main park office, you will cross over the dam on a narrow one-lane road. Follow the signs heading north to Westside Campground Loop Road, and follow that road to the park office. Across from the office parking lot is a very clean, well-equipped comfort station with showers.

At Sumner Lake State Park, piñon, juniper, and mesquite trees and yucca cover the hills surrounding the lake. Common varieties of cacti include cholla and prickly pear. Cottonwood trees grow along the Pecos River area, which is the shadiest area of the park. Fishing reports for the lake vary by season, but the target species are mostly warm-water varieties, including largemouth bass, white bass, crappie, and channel catfish. From time to time, you will see mule deer and pronghorn antelope, and there are signs warning of mountain lions along the river, so beware.

At capacity, the reservoir covers around 4,900 water acres; the park covers 6,700

## :: Ratings

BEAUTY: ★ ★ ★ ★
PRIVACY: ★ ★ ★
SPACIOUSNESS: ★ ★ ★
QUIET: ★ ★ ★ ★
SECURITY: ★ ★ ★ ★ ★
CLEANLINESS: ★ ★ ★ ★ ★

acres. The Pecos River flows into the reservoir at the north end of the lake and continues as it flows out at the spillway dam. The dam was built in 1939 to prevent the low-lying areas along the Pecos River from flooding during the monsoon season. The lake is a beautiful deep blue and offers many opportunities for water sports, such as boating, canoeing, kayaking, windsurfing, waterskiing, and swimming. Life preservers are mandatory while enjoying the lake. There are swimming areas around the lake, but some areas may be off-limits to swimming; inquire at the office or ask the park rangers for approved swimming areas. In recent years, New Mexico has been fighting drought, and the lake was down during my visits in the fall of 2013.

### WEST SIDE CAMPGROUNDS

Pecos and Mesquite Campgrounds are the RV loops to the west of the park office, but if you turn right onto the dirt road just south of the park office, there are four nonelectric campsites, and between them and the lake are large areas for primitive camping all the way south until you get to the overlook loop. There is not much shade close to the lakeside, but there are some juniper and piñon trees that sit back from the lake under which you can pitch your tent. Spots of sparse grass provide places to set up your tent. These sites are considered primitive, so there's no picnic table, just trash bins. Needless to say, it would

## :: Key Information

**ADDRESS:** 32 Lakeview Ln., Sumner Lake, NM 88119

**OPERATED BY:** New Mexico State Parks

**CONTACT:** 575-355-2541; **www.emnrd.state.nm.us/SPD /sumnerlakestatepark.html**

**OPEN:** *West Side Campgrounds* year-round; *East Side Campground* May 1– end of Sept.

**SITES:** 50 developed sites, plus primitive and group sites

**SITE AMENITIES:** Developed sites have parking space, picnic table, and platform grill.

**ASSIGNMENT:** First come, first served or reserve at **reserveamerica.com** or 877-664-7787.

**REGISTRATION:** At visitor center or self-registration on-site

**FACILITIES:** Restrooms, showers, vault toilets, dump station, visitor center, boat dock, playground

**PARKING:** At each site

**FEE:** $8 primitive, $10 nonelectric, $14 with electric or sewage hookup, $18 with electric and sewage hookups; $5 day-use fee per vehicle

**ELEVATION:** 4,300 feet

**RESTRICTIONS**

■ **Pets:** On 10-foot leash; take precautionary measures against predators.

■ **Fires:** No ground fires permitted; charcoal grills permitted

■ **Alcohol:** At campsites only; zero tolerance while boating

■ **Other:** Quiet hours 10 p.m.–8 a.m.; 14-day stay limit

---

be helpful to have a sun shelter here. At the entrance to the west campgrounds, The Fisherman's Hideaway bar, restaurant, and store provides ice, groceries, and package goods.

### EAST SIDE CAMPGROUND

On the east side of the lake there are more opportunities for primitive camping but fewer trees under which to camp. As you head north on East Campground Road, turn onto Beaver Shore Road and you'll find many primitive sites all the way to East Side Campground. There you will find restrooms and nonelectric sites. Slightly north of East Side Campground you will find areas where the trees are a little more plentiful for shade.

### SHADY SIDE CAMPGROUND

Westside River Road leads down to the bottom of the dam and Shady Side Campground.

Under a mix of Russian olive, salt cedar, and cottonwood trees, you will find all the shade you'll need to enjoy great camping along the Pecos River, right below the spillway. The sites are dispersed on this side, but you will find soft grassy areas to set up your tent. The campground has a vault toilet, trash bins, and a pay station, but there are no water spigots here. For water, visit the lakeside campgrounds. Even though you are camping at a primitive site, you are still allowed to go up to the lake and use the park facilities, including the showers. Since the camping is dispersed, you may find space can get a little tight on a busy weekend.

### RACCOON CAMPGROUND

Just east of the dam, the access road leads down to Raccoon Campground. You'll find plenty of shade here. A few sites are developed, but there are also a number of grassy and shady areas for primitive camping. Raccoon Campground also has a vault toilet, trash bins, and a pay station. Raccoon is a little wider than Shady Side and can accommodate more camps, but it can also get crowded on busy weekends.

## Nearby Attraction

### FORT SUMNER, NEW MEXICO:
### Burial Place of Billy the Kid

The town and outpost of Fort Sumner began in 1862 as a US Army Post built to detain Navajo and Mescalero Apache Indians. By 1868, the fort was abandoned and the Navajo and Mescalero Apaches returned to their homelands.

In 1869, a wealthy cattle baron, Lucien Maxwell, purchased the abandoned Fort Sumner outpost and converted one of the buildings to a hacienda. Maxwell retired, sold his holdings in 1870, and died in 1875. The Fort Sumner property was deeded to his son, Pete Maxwell. William Bonney, aka Billy the Kid, visited Fort Sumner frequently, was good friends with Pete Maxwell, and courted Pete's younger sister, Paulita.

At the end of the Lincoln County war, Billy was locked up in the jail in Lincoln and was to be hung on May 13, 1881. On April 28, he broke out of jail, killing two deputies. A few months after the jailbreak, Sheriff Pat Garrett caught wind that Billy was in Fort Sumner, so he headed there to question Pete Maxwell. Around midnight on July 14, 1881, Pat Garrett was at Pete Maxwell's hacienda when Billy walked into the room. Garrett reached for his pistol and fired twice. The first bullet pierced Billy right above the heart.

Billy the Kid was buried in the Fort Sumner Military Cemetery between his two outlaw friends, Tom O'Folliard and Charlie Bowdre, killed earlier that same year. The graves of Lucien and Pete Maxwell are also in this cemetery. In 1889 and 1904, the Pecos River floods washed away all the grave markers. For more than 20 years Billy's grave was left unmarked, but some old-timers were able to reliably determine where his grave was located. In 1932, funds were raised to provide a tombstone for the three outlaws. The headstone has been chipped over and over from souvenir hunters. In 1940, a footstone was donated to the cemetery. The footstone was stolen in 1950 and found 26 years later in Texas. After its return, the footstone was stolen again in 1981 but found in California a few days later and returned. The village constructed a steel cage to protect the gravesite and preserve the chipped headstone. After all this effort, on June 16, 2012, vandals broke into the cage at night and tipped over the headstone. Billy's footstone is now secured in a welded steel cage (oddly similar to a jail cell) to discourage vandalism.

The gravesite is located at the **Old Fort Sumner Museum.** The museum is well worth the $5 admission. You can spend as much time as you wish viewing and photographing the rich history of the Old West. From downtown Fort Sumner, follow US 60/84 east; turn right (south) on Billy the Kid Drive (NM 272) and follow it 3 miles to the museum at the intersection of NM 272 and NM 212. The museum will be on the right, and the cemetery entrance is just past the museum entrance. For more information, call 575-355-2942.

The Billy the Kid Museum, located 2 miles east of downtown Fort Sumner at 1435 East Sumner Avenue, is also a worthwhile attraction. Admission is also $5, and you can load up on Billy the Kid souvenirs at the gift shop. For more information, visit **billythe kidmuseumfortsumner.com.**

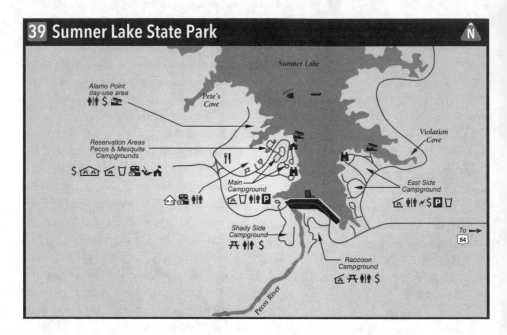

**39** Sumner Lake State Park

## :: Getting There

From I-40 at Santa Rosa, drive south on US 84 for 32 miles. Turn west on NM 203 and drive 5.5 miles to Sumner Lake State Park.

**GPS COORDINATES**  N34° 36.937'  W104° 22.668'

# Southwestern
# New Mexico

# 40

# El Morro National Monument

*Follow in the path of ancient native peoples and the Spanish conquistadors and camp at this shady little campground on a sloping hill.*

**O**n the hunt for off-the-beaten-path, peaceful, and remote tent-camping areas, my wife, Susan, and I stumbled upon this quaint little campground that has it all. Ancient native people and the Spanish conquistadors must have agreed—they camped here as well.

El Morro Campground doesn't even have a name, so I nicknamed it Camp El Mo. Tiny Camp El Mo is to the left off the access road on the way to El Morro Visitor Center. It's well equipped, brand new in appearance, and sparkling clean. The camp is just one small loop, and the compactness and tight turns prevent RVs and fifth-wheel trailers from accessing it. Plus, most parking areas would not hold much more than one passenger vehicle. I was amused when I read some of the reviews by these RV drivers, aggravated that they were unable to utilize the camp. I imagine that pop-up campers and cab-over campers would be able to squeeze into the campground successfully.

## :: Ratings

BEAUTY: ★ ★ ★ ★
PRIVACY: ★ ★ ★
SPACIOUSNESS: ★ ★ ★
QUIET: ★ ★ ★ ★ ★
SECURITY: ★ ★ ★
CLEANLINESS: ★ ★ ★ ★ ★

Although there's no fee, Camp El Mo does have a bulletin board that requires all users to register. There are water spigots between sites 1 and 2 and 6 and 7. Nearly all sites have a trash bin, and at the vault toilet, there are varmint-proof trash bins and recycle bins. The low-odor vault toilets were recently constructed. Directly across from the toilets is ADA-accessible site 5, with a large concrete pad; this site also has an ADA picnic table, plus the ADA raised fire pit.

All sites have adequate shade, provided by piñon, cedar, and juniper trees, but the climate here is too arid to allow for any grassy areas. From the top to the bottom of the loop, there is a slight declining slope, which provides good runoff when it rains, plus a commanding view of the El Morro National Monument and Inscription Rock.

Be sure to take some time to explore the monument. Your first stop should be the visitor center to check out the 15-minute video presentation, maps, and information available to aid in understanding the geologic, historic, and cultural significance of this monument. The Zuni Indians called Inscription Rock A'ts'ina, or "place of writings on rock." The Spaniards called it El Morro, or "the headland." The magnificently preserved ruins atop A'ts'ina were built in approximately 1275, and it's estimated that they were occupied for only 75 years. The inscriptions were made first by the Native

## :: Key Information

**ADDRESS:** El Morro National Monument, HC61, Box 43, Ramah, NM 87321-9603

**OPERATED BY:** National Park Service

**CONTACT:** 585-783-4226; **nps.gov/elmo**

**OPEN:** Year-round, except Christmas and New Year's Days

**SITES:** 9

**SITE AMENITIES:** Parking space, picnic table, tent box, fire ring

**ASSIGNMENT:** First come, first served

**REGISTRATION:** Self-registration on-site

**FACILITIES:** Vault toilets, visitor center

**PARKING:** At each site

**FEE:** None

**ELEVATION:** 7,191 feet

**RESTRICTIONS**

■ **Pets:** On 6-foot leash; take precautionary measures against predators.

■ **Fires:** In fire rings only; charcoal grills permitted; check with Forest Service office and postings on the camp bulletin board for restrictions.

■ **Alcohol:** At campsites only

■ **Other:** Quiet hours 10 p.m.– 8 a.m.; 14-day stay limit

tribes, and then much later by Spaniards, namely Don Juan de Onate on April 16, 1605. One of the attractions of Inscription Rock in times past was a life-sustaining pool of water at the base of the rock. That same pool exists today, and this is where de Onate's mark can be found.

### Nearby Attraction

At the **Wild Spirit Wolf Sanctuary** visitors learn about wolves, wolf-dogs, and other related species, as well as our ecosystem and how we all play a part in it. The sanctuary is open Tuesday–Sunday, and tours are available at 11 a.m. and 12:30, 2, and 3:30 p.m. Admission is $7 for adults, $6 for seniors, and $4 for children; kids under 7 admitted free. For directions and more information, visit **wildspiritwolfsanctuary.org** or call 505-775-3304.

Just across the street from Wild Spirit Wolf Sanctuary is a beautiful primitive campground. It's shaded and close enough to the sanctuary to hear the wolves singing all night. Each site includes a picnic table and fire pit, and there are fully equipped shower houses. Cost is $15 per night, and propane grills can be rented for another $15 per night. To make reservations, call 505-775-3304.

To get there, take I-40 to Grants. At Exit 81, turn left onto NM 53 and go about 50 miles. About 2 miles past El Morro, look for a sign for Mountainview & Pine Hill. Turn left onto BIA 125 and go 8 miles. Turn right onto gravel road BIA 120. Wild Spirit Wolf Sanctuary is 4 miles down on the left.

## :: Getting There

From Grants, take I-40 to Exit 81 and go southwest on NM 53 for 42 miles. The turn-off for the monument is on the south side of NM 53. Look for the sign that marks the entrance.

**GPS COORDINATES**     N35° 2.199'   W108° 20.275'

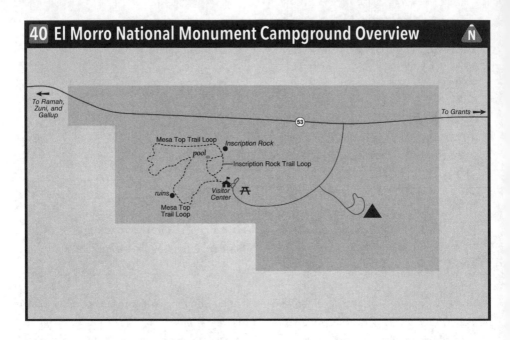

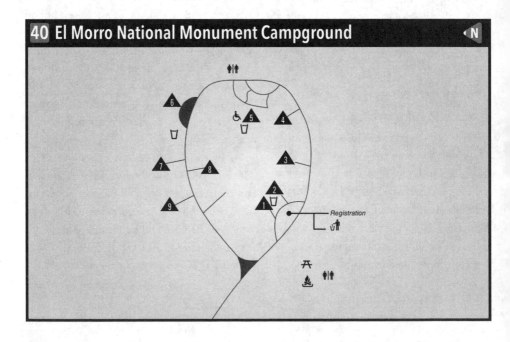

# 41

# Joe Skeen Campground

*From Joe Skeen, you can explore La Ventana Arch, the Narrows, and El Malpais lava bed.*

**W**ithin the confines of the El Malpais National Conservation area are several geologic attractions. The name El Malpais is the Spanish term meaning "the badlands," which is appropriate because of the extremely barren and dramatic lava field that covers much of the park's area. From the time you leave I-40, you will begin to see the large lava bed, which extends 35 miles and ends about 18 miles south of La Ventana Natural Arch.

Joe Skeen Campground lacks the beauty of many of the campgrounds in this book; however, the area around this camp is teeming with magnificent natural beauty. Joe Skeen is a no-frills roadside campground. Even though it is a roadside camp, most evenings will be quiet with very little traffic. There is no water, so you will need to carry in your own, or you can stop at the BLM office (2 miles to the north) from 9 a.m. to 4 p.m., and they will allow you to fill one 5-gallon water container.

The campground is well equipped for primitive camping. Joe Skeen is void of any trees, so shade is rather scarce, but sheltered picnic tables provide a welcome escape from the hot New Mexico sun. A four-wheel-drive road goes off to the east, and there are sites for camping along that road, but you should clear it with the BLM office first.

Several good hiking areas are nearby, but beware of rattlesnakes—this is the ideal environment for them. Check with the visitor center for trail information.

There are also several local sights to visit in this area. The most interesting is La Ventana Natural Arch, the second-largest natural arch in New Mexico. It's located 17 miles south of Joe Skeen Campground on NM 117. La Ventana means "the window" in Spanish. The trail to the arch is not a hike at all; it's more like a casual stroll. Since the arch faces southwest, the best time to photograph it is in early to late afternoon. La Ventana Arch is an incredible sightseeing stop that you will not want to miss. The drive from the arch south toward Quemado features spectacular cliffs on the east side of the road. The area is called The Narrows, and it too is a very pretty and worthwhile excursion.

A little more than a mile north of the Joe Skeen Campground, you'll find the dirt Sandstone Bluff Road, located on the west side of NM 117. At the end of the road is a loop where you can park. Walk out to the edge of the sandstone bluff for incredible views overlooking the lava field.

## :: Ratings

BEAUTY: ★ ★ ★
PRIVACY: ★ ★ ★
SPACIOUSNESS: ★ ★ ★
QUIET: ★ ★ ★ ★ ★
SECURITY: ★ ★ ★ ★ ★
CLEANLINESS: ★ ★ ★ ★ ★

## :: Key Information

**ADDRESS:** El Malpais National Conservation Area, P.O. Box 846, Grants, NM 87020

**OPERATED BY:** Bureau of Land Management

**CONTACT:** 505-280-2918 (ranger station) or 585-783-4226; **blm.gov**

**OPEN:** Year-round; ranger station open daily 9 a.m.–4 p.m.

**SITES:** 10

**SITE AMENITIES:** Parking space, picnic table, fire ring

**ASSIGNMENT:** First come, first served

**REGISTRATION:** Self-registration on-site

**FACILITIES:** Vault toilets; bring water.

**PARKING:** At each site

**FEE:** None

**ELEVATION:** 6,686 feet

**RESTRICTIONS**

■ **Pets:** On 6-foot leash; take precautionary measures against predators.

■ **Fires:** In fire rings only; charcoal grills permitted; check with BLM office for restrictions; bring your own firewood.

■ **Alcohol:** At campsites only

■ **Other:** Quiet hours 10 p.m.–8 a.m.; 14-day stay limit

The Lava field here is similar to the lava fields near the Valley of Fires Campground (see page 116). The lava is the same type as found in the Hawaiian Islands, pahoehoe and a'a. The lava field begins just south of the I-40 exit and stretches 35 miles south. The vent associated with this lava flow can be visited off NM 53, at the Banderas Crater. Follow recommended guidelines for hiking the lava fields. Durable footwear, such as hard-soled hiking boots, is highly recommended.

Junction Cave is a 3,000-foot-long lava tube, just one of many lava tube caves in the park. To venture underground, and for your safety, the El Malpais visitor center provides a mandatory free caving permit. Caves currently available for access include Junction, Xenolith, Big Skylight, and Giant Ice. Junction and Xenolith Caves are in the El Calderon Area, and Big Skylight and Giant Ice Caves are in the Big Tubes Area. For your safety while caving, take several light sources and wear boots, a hat, gloves, and protective clothing.

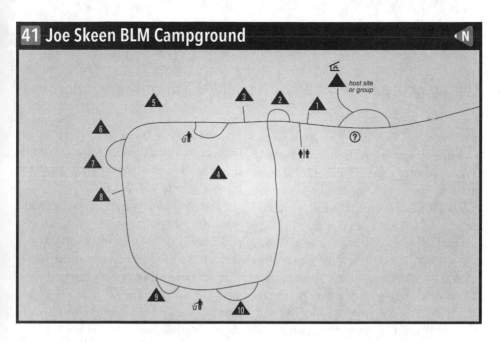

## :: Getting There

From Grants, take I-40 to Exit 89 and turn right (south) on NM 117. Follow NM 117 for 11 miles to the campground.

**GPS COORDINATES** N34° 58.254' W107° 48.620'

# 42

# Pancho Villa State Park

*This 49-acre park boasts indescribably beautiful cactus gardens.*

**P**ancho Villa State Park features a campground with historical significance. This is the exact location of Camp Furlong, one of the two sites raided in 1916 by Mexican Revolutionary General Francisco "Pancho" Villa. Villa raided the camp and the tiny settlement of Columbus, a few blocks to the north. Twenty-four Americans were killed in the raid. The town of Columbus had 400 residents and was left a fiery rubble at battle's end. This is the only site since the War of 1812 in which the United States has been invaded by armed foreign troops. Scattered throughout the grounds of the park are ruins of this once-bustling U.S. Army 13th Calvary camp that housed 350 troops.

The $1.8 million museum was dedicated in 2006 and remains free to campers. It contains a full-size replica Curtiss JN-3 "Jenny" airplane used by the 1st Aero Squadron, a 1915 Dodge touring car riddled with bullet holes from the raid, historical artifacts, and military weapons and ribbons. The first armored tank ever used by the U.S. Army in battle stands sentinel outside the facility. The airfield was located across US 11 from Camp Furlong. The pursuit of Villa

by General John "Black Jack" Pershing was unsuccessful but historic. It was the first time aircraft and battle tanks were used in combat prior to World War I.

Indescribably beautiful cactus gardens are scattered throughout the entire 49-acre park. The cacti bloom from early March through the end of May, an excellent time to visit. Six ruins are worthy of photographs, so do not forget your camera. Coote's Hill is the predominant landmark of the park. It was there that, under cover of darkness, the Villista raiders scouted around the north side of the hill to attack the camp and the town of Columbus. Today, Coote's Hill is beautiful, and cacti of every species thrive on the hillsides. There was a terrible freeze a few years ago, but some of the cacti are coming back. A paved walkway leads to the hill's crest. You can see 100 miles on a clear day, and view nearby Palomas, Mexico, 3 miles to the south.

This Chihuahuan Desert park boasts 79 developed sites for RVs, a small area for tents, plus three tent sites (C1–C3) on the west side of Coote's Hill. A new addition for tents is located in the RV campground in the far south end of the park. The main tent area to the east of Coote's Hill has a windbreak of cottonwood and willow trees, which helps to partition the tent area from the RV area. The main tent area is perfectly level, with several picnic tables and one shade shelter. It is surrounded by cactus gardens and within walking distance of everything in the park. Tent campers can choose from all primitive

## :: Ratings

BEAUTY: ★ ★ ★
PRIVACY: ★ ★ ★
SPACIOUSNESS: ★ ★ ★
QUIET: ★ ★ ★ ★
SECURITY: ★ ★ ★ ★ ★
CLEANLINESS: ★ ★ ★ ★ ★

## :: Key Information

**ADDRESS:** Junction of Hwys. 9 and 11, Columbus, NM 88029

**OPERATED BY:** New Mexico State Parks

**CONTACT:** 575-531-2711; www.emnrd.state.nm.us/SPD /panchovillastatepark.html

**OPEN:** Year-round

**SITES:** 79 developed sites (75 with electric), plus primitive sites

**SITE AMENITIES:** Parking space, picnic table; developed sites have sun shade over a picnic table and fire ring.

**ASSIGNMENT:** Sites 3–8 can be reserved at **reserveamerica.com** or 877-664-7787; all other sites are first come, first served.

**REGISTRATION:** Self-registration on-site without a reservation; with reservation, follow instructions on website and print receipt of reservation for check-in.

**FACILITIES:** Restrooms, showers, dump station, visitor center, playground

**PARKING:** At each site

**FEE:** $8 primitive, $10 nonelectric, $14 with electric or sewage hookup, $18 with electric and sewage hookups; $5 day-use fee per vehicle

**ELEVATION:** 4,064 feet

**RESTRICTIONS**

■ **Pets:** On 6-foot leash; take precautionary measures against rattlesnakes.

■ **Fires:** In fire rings only; charcoal grills permitted; check with campground host, park office, and postings on the camp bulletin board for restrictions.

■ **Alcohol:** At campsites only

■ **Other:** Quiet hours 10 p.m.–8 a.m.; 14-day stay limit

---

sites. No specific numbers are assigned to the undeveloped tent areas; they're on a first-come, first-serve basis. Tent campers can also select a developed site if they want a sun shelter over the picnic table. The rangers, volunteer camp hosts, and museum staff are very helpful and friendly.

Greasewood and mesquite trees dot the park. There is no firewood gathering, so bring your own. Portable fire rings are available for the asking. The modern pressurized water system delivers treated water. Two modern, spotlessly clean comfort stations have sinks, flush toilets, and warm-water showers.

Cottontail rabbits inhabit this park in great numbers. Various bird species abound, and quail scurrying around the camp are a common sight.

Snowbirds are attracted to this park during winter months, when daytime temperatures rarely plummet below the 50°F range. Summers may exceed 110°F, and there are no nearby ponds, streams, or swimming pools in which to cool off. Spring and fall are excellent seasons to visit but can be windy. Campground roads are gravel, and the wind can generate a dusty camping experience.

Columbus has 700 residents, several cafés, a grocery store, two service stations, and a museum located in the former train depot. The sleepy little border town of Palomas, Mexico, is 3 miles to the south. Shopping, restaurants, and medical and dental clinics are plentiful in Palomas, but due to the upsurge in drug cartel violence, border towns are high-risk places and visiting is discouraged. Proof of US citizenship is required to get back across the border, and contraband searches are performed regularly by the U.S. Border Patrol upon reentry.

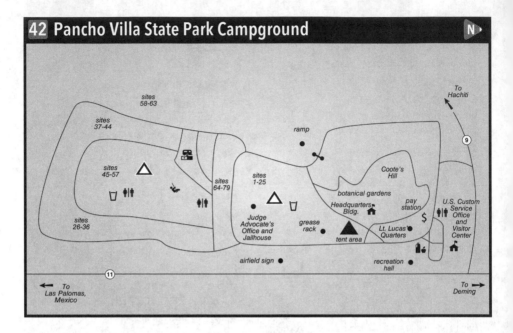

## 42 Pancho Villa State Park Campground

sites
58-63

sites
37-44

ramp

sites
45-57

Coote's
Hill

sites
64-79

sites
1-25

botanical gardens

pay
station

sites
26-36

Headquarters
Bldg.

U.S. Custom
Service
Office
and
Visitor
Center

Judge
Advocate's
Office and
Jailhouse

grease
rack

tent area

Lt. Lucas'
Quarters

airfield sign

recreation
hall

To
Las Palomas,
Mexico

To
Deming

To
Hachiti

## :: Getting There

From Deming, drive 35 miles south on US 11 to the intersection of US 9. Turn right
(west) on US 9, and the park entrance is on south side.

**GPS COORDINATES**   N31° 49.467'   W107° 38.433'

# 43

# Water Canyon Campground

*A surprisingly pretty getaway tucked in a small box canyon*

**W**ater Canyon Campground is a surprisingly scenic getaway tucked in a small box canyon just 22 miles southwest of Socorro. It is an ideal family campground, with bicycle trails and one hiking trail that leads to the top of the canyon.

The Magdalena Mountains are home to black bears, coyotes, mountain lions, bobcats, deer, elk, turkeys, bald eagles, and several varieties of hawks. The cliff walls of Water Canyon provide habitat for peregrine falcons and many other varieties of birds. Hummingbirds love this canyon too.

The entry road is dirt and gravel (so quite dusty), with a few tight turns. The campground loop is also tight, so you will see few RVs at this camp. No campground host is assigned here, but the Forest Service patrols occasionally, as does the New Mexico Department of Game and Fish.

The forest provides good shade, with ponderosa pine, alligator juniper, piñon, and cedar trees. Most days are warm; it is an ideal campground for spring and fall, but summers can be hot. You'll find plenty of downed firewood here. This canyon can get very dry, and campfire restrictions can go into effect with little notice, so calling ahead is advisable. There's no water here, so bring your own, and make sure you have plenty for both drinking and dousing your fire.

Each campsite has a fire ring and picnic table with adequate parking. There is no grass, and the ground can be quite rocky, so bring a high-quality ground pad. Most sites are small, and there is little privacy, with the exception of trees between the sites. Two modern wheelchair-accessible vault toilets are available; one is situated at the entrance and the other is on the end loop with varmint-proof trash bins. If the trash bins are full, you must pack out your trash. This campground is kept extremely clean by campers.

Just past the campground entrance is the group camp, which is used for overflow if it is not reserved. The group camp has one modern wheelchair-accessible vault toilet and a large shelter.

The large grassy picnic area is located at the bottom of the hill before you reach the main campground. The picnic area has a modern wheelchair-accessible vault toilet, a large group shelter, several pedestal grills, and a small stream. The stream is usually dry unless it rains or there's snowmelt.

Water Canyon's nearest supply center is the town of Magdalena. While driving down Forest Service Road 235, you may see large herds of pronghorn antelope. This road is open range, with little fencing, so be careful. Two other small campgrounds, Beartrap and Hughes Mill, are nearby. Combined, these two camps have eight sites.

## :: Ratings

BEAUTY: ★ ★ ★ ★
PRIVACY: ★
SPACIOUSNESS: ★
QUIET: ★ ★ ★
SECURITY: ★ ★
CLEANLINESS: ★ ★ ★ ★ ★

## :: Key Information

**ADDRESS:** Cibola National Forest, Magdalena Ranger District, P.O. Box 45, Magdalena, NM 87825

**OPERATED BY:** U.S. Department of Agriculture

**CONTACT:** 505-854-2281; www.fs.usda.gov/cibola

**OPEN:** April 1–late fall

**SITES:** 12

**SITE AMENITIES:** Parking space, picnic table, fire ring

**ASSIGNMENT:** First come, first served

**REGISTRATION:** Self-registration on-site

**FACILITIES:** Vault toilets

**PARKING:** At each site

**FEE:** None

**ELEVATION:** 6,926 feet

**RESTRICTIONS**

■ **Pets:** On 6-foot leash; take precautionary measures against predators.

■ **Fires:** In fire rings only; charcoal grills permitted; check with Forest Service office and postings on the camp bulletin board for restrictions.

■ **Alcohol:** At campsites only

■ **Other:** Quiet hours 10 p.m.–8 a.m.; 14-day stay limit

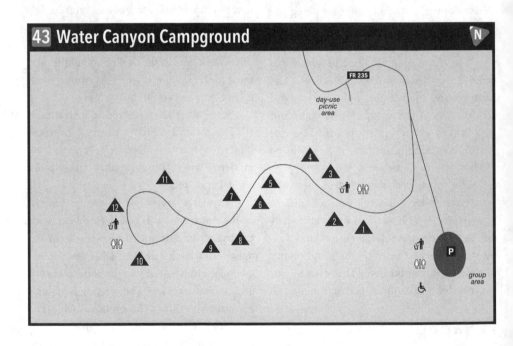

**43 Water Canyon Campground**

## :: Getting There

From Socorro, drive west on NM 60 for 16 miles, and then turn south on FR 235 at the Water Canyon sign and go 4.5 miles to the camp.

**GPS COORDINATES**   N34° 1.455'   W107° 8.017'

# 44

# Datil Well Campground

*This comfortable little camp is a historic stop along the old Magdalena cattle trail.*

**D**atil Well is named for the town of Datil, 1 mile to the west. This is the location of one of 15 water wells spaced 10 miles apart along the old Magdalena Cattle Trail. This trail was established in January of 1885 and stretched 120 miles from Springerville, Arizona, to Magdalena, New Mexico.

The Atchison, Topeka, and Santa Fe Railway completed its line from Magdalena to Socorro, and ranchers began driving their livestock to Magdalena for shipment. 1919 was the peak year of use of the trail, when 150,000 sheep and 21,667 cattle made the journey. The trail was set aside by the U.S. Department of the Interior in 1918 as a result of the Endangered Grazing Homestead Act.

The campground is scenic and shaded with a mix of juniper, cedar, and piñon trees. Most campsites are rather small, but plenty of trees between the sites provide adequate privacy. Five water spigots are spread equally throughout the campground, delivering treated water from the same source that was used in the cattle drives. Three modern vault toilets are scattered conveniently throughout the campground, and one is wheelchair accessible. There is a trove of information and brochures at the pay station building.

No special area exists for tent campers, but all sites are ideal for tents. The ground is level, with a mix of fine gravel and sand; there's no grass. Sites on the outside of the loop provide more shade and separation from the other sites and come with a view of the surrounding San Augustin Plains. Keep in mind that RVs do use this campground and generators are allowed. A camp host is assigned here from April until November.

The Bureau of Land Management manages this campground well, providing each campsite with a small armful of wood for a campfire. There may be a large stack of firewood available for your use, but please leave what you do not use. A short hike from the perimeter of the campground will supply enough firewood for resourceful campers.

Three miles of hiking trails meander throughout the nearby woodlands. Hiking trails are for foot traffic only; no bicycles or motorized vehicles are permitted access. Winter snows provide excellent snowshoeing and cross-country skiing. All trails range from easy to moderate, and three overlooks provide views of Crosby Canyon and the San Augustin Plains.

Heavy rains have blessed this area with green grasses and many species of wildflowers. You will see occasional deer and coyotes,

## :: Ratings

BEAUTY: ★ ★ ★
PRIVACY: ★ ★ ★ ★
SPACIOUSNESS: ★ ★
QUIET: ★ ★ ★ ★
SECURITY: ★ ★ ★ ★ ★
CLEANLINESS: ★ ★ ★ ★ ★

## :: Key Information

**ADDRESS:** Bureau of Land Management, Soccoro Field Office, 901 US 85, Soccoro, NM 87113

**OPERATED BY:** Bureau of Land Management

**CONTACT:** 575-835-0412; **blm.gov**

**OPEN:** Year-round

**SITES:** 22

**SITE AMENITIES:** Parking space, picnic table, trash bin, fire ring, grill; some with shelters

**ASSIGNMENT:** First come, first served

**REGISTRATION:** Self-registration on-site

**FACILITIES:** Restrooms

**PARKING:** At each site

**FEE:** $5

**ELEVATION:** 7,441 feet

**RESTRICTIONS**

■ **Pets:** On 6-foot leash; take precautionary measures against predators.

■ **Fires:** In fire rings only; charcoal grills permitted

■ **Alcohol:** At campsites only

■ **Other:** Quiet hours 10 p.m.–8 a.m.; 7-day stay limit

and many varieties of reptiles, including several species of rattlesnakes. Black bears, bobcats, and mountain lions also inhabit this area. Be on the lookout for herds of pronghorn antelope; they are abundant in the San Augustin Plains area. And bring the hummingbird feeder; the broad-tailed variety is abundant here.

Summer temperatures can soar close to 90°F here, but evenings cool off to the mid-50s. Summer rains arrive almost daily with the New Mexico monsoon season, so be careful and take cover if lightning is present. Winter can bring more than a foot of snow, providing an excellent experience for adventurous campers. Water hydrants are turned off in November, but water is available in Datil.

Fifteen miles east of Datil, a series of 27 radio telescopes, spread in a Y pattern across the San Augustin Plains, comprise the Very Large Array (VLA). The VLA has been used by more astronomers than any other radio telescope worldwide.

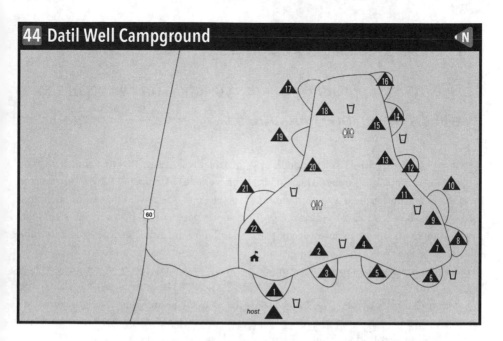

**44 Datil Well Campground**

## :: Getting There

From Datil, at the junction of US 60 and NM 12, follow US 60 1 mile to the northwest. Turn left at campground sign.

**GPS COORDINATES**   N34° 9.250'   W107° 51.488'

# 45

# Pinon Campground

*This lovely campground provides commanding views of the lake and surrounding mountains.*

**P**inon Campground is shaded by piñon, cedar, and juniper trees. This lovely campground provides commanding views of the lake and surrounding mountains. Due to its location away from the lake, there is less traffic in this campground and it's more peaceful than nearby Juniper Campground.

Pinon Camp is divided into two separate areas; the road to the right leads to a huge group campground with several group shelters. The road to the left leads to the individual campsites. Twenty-two individual sites, numbered 37–59 are located on the left loop. The sites on the outside of the loop have more space between them, and there is some privacy between the sites, thanks to the trees. Two sites are designated for disabled campers. Two composting toilets are at each end of the campground, and trash bins and water spigots are located next to the toilet buildings. The water is potable.

The ground is rocky, but most sites provide a gravel tent box. The road is crushed gravel and can get quite dusty. By setting your tent back in the trees, your sleeping quarters will escape the dust clouds of passing vehicles. Campsite tables are located too close to the road, and traffic passing at a snail's pace can coat your meals with dust.

There are no electrical sites here, and the design of this campground is predominantly intended for tent camping. There were no RVs here during my stay. The parking is not conducive to RVs, and most opt for the Juniper Campground across the highway.

Forest Service employees work constantly at Pinon, and the Catron County Sheriff's Department and Forest Service law enforcement officers keep a close eye on the campground, so it is secure. You should bring your own firewood or gather wood near the El Caso Campground areas. A campground host sells wood for $5 per bundle. El Caso Campgrounds are nondeveloped campgrounds located at the east end of Quemado Lake, 0.5 mile east of Pinon Campground. These areas are nestled in a valley surrounded by ponderosa pine and cottonwood trees, which offer excellent shade. Camping is free there.

## :: Ratings

BEAUTY: ★ ★ ★
PRIVACY: ★ ★
SPACIOUSNESS: ★ ★ ★
QUIET: ★ ★ ★ ★
SECURITY: ★ ★ ★ ★ ★
CLEANLINESS: ★ ★ ★ ★ ★

## :: Key Information

**ADDRESS:** Gila National Forest, Quemado Ranger District, P.O. Box 158, Quemado, NM 87829

**OPERATED BY:** U.S. Department of Agriculture

**CONTACT:** 575-773-4678; www.fs.usda.gov/gila

**OPEN:** May 1–Sept. 30; lower loop open until Nov. 14 but without water; toilets remain open.

**SITES:** 22

**SITE AMENITIES:** Parking space, picnic table, pedestal grill, fire ring

**ASSIGNMENT:** First come, first served

**REGISTRATION:** Self-registration on-site

**FACILITIES:** Vault toilets

**PARKING:** At each site

**FEE:** $10

**ELEVATION:** 7,862 feet

**RESTRICTIONS**

■ **Pets:** On 6-foot leash; take precautionary measures against predators.

■ **Fires:** In fire rings and pedestal grills only; charcoal grills permitted

■ **Alcohol:** At campsites only

■ **Other:** Quiet hours 10 p.m.–8 a.m.; 15-day stay limit

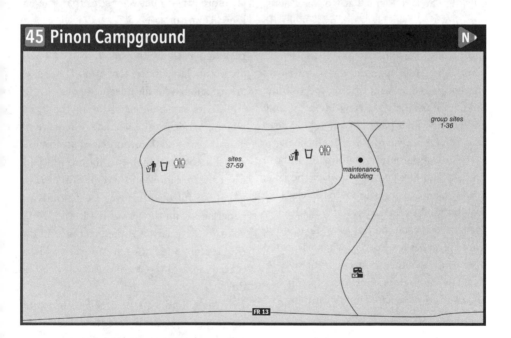

## :: Getting There

West of Quemado, take NM 32 south 14.2 miles to the Quemado Lake/NM 103 sign. At the sign, turn left onto NM 103 and go 4 miles to Forest Service Road 13 (gravel). Continue straight on FR 13 for 1.4 miles to the campground sign. Turn left into campground.

**GPS COORDINATES**   N34° 5.675'   W108° 26.218'

# 46

# Juniper Campground

*Juniper Campground is the closest camp to Quemado Lake, which offers excellent fishing.*

**For those** who love lake camping, Quemado Lake offers several good campgrounds. The closest camp to the lake is Juniper Campground, but this is not lakeshore camping. The fishing here can be excellent, with rainbow and lake trout the most common catches, along with the occasional tiger muskie. The lake is small at 130 water acres but provides two boat ramps. Quemado Lake is excellent for canoeing, kayaking, and rafting. Personal flotation devices are mandatory while upon the water, and boats are required to travel at trolling speeds only; this is a no-wake lake. New Mexico Game and Fish wardens patrol frequently, so keep your fishing license with you at all times.

The campground sits atop a knoll above the lake and gives partial views of the lake; however, most campsite views of the lake are obscured by trees. Several trails lead to the lake, less than 100 feet away. Road noise from Forest Service Road 13, which is located up the hill from the camp, is a problem here.

The campground provides 36 spaces: Sites 1–18 are designated for RV camping and are on a separate loop from the tent area. These sites are arranged in six clusters, with three campsites in each cluster. Each site has electric and water hookups. While there is privacy between clusters, there is no privacy between sites in each cluster. The tent area, sites 19–36, is quite large and provides far more privacy between sites than the RV loop. Unfortunately, a few RVs will camp here, but there are plenty of sites where the parking spaces are too small for RVs. There are no hookups in the tent area. Three sites are designated for disabled campers.

Tents can be erected under the trees, which provide excellent shade. There are no grassy areas, and the ground is rocky in some spots, so bring a high-quality ground pad. Most sites are level, and several sites provide a tent box filled with gravel. Dust clouds are generated from the gravel road, even when vehicles drive slowly. A picnic table and fire ring are provided at each campsite and are placed close to the road; mealtimes can be dusty.

You'll find two new self-composting toilets, one at the loop entrance and the other at the end of the loop. Trash bins and pressurized water spigots are located near the toilets. Two other spigots, one pressurized and one hand-pump spigot, are located on the loop. The water is treated. Bathing, cleaning pots and pans, and cleaning fish are strictly prohibited at the spigot areas. Showers are not provided at

## :: Ratings

BEAUTY: ★ ★ ★ ★
PRIVACY: ★ ★
SPACIOUSNESS: ★ ★ ★
QUIET: ★ ★
SECURITY: ★ ★ ★ ★ ★
CLEANLINESS: ★ ★ ★ ★ ★

## :: Key Information

**ADDRESS:** Gila National Forest, Quemado Ranger District, P.O. Box 158, Quemado, NM 87829

**OPERATED BY:** U.S. Department of Agriculture

**CONTACT:** 575-773-4678; www.fs.usda.gov/gila

**OPEN:** May 1–Nov. 1

**SITES:** 36

**SITE AMENITIES:** Parking space, picnic table, fire ring; several with gravel tent boxes and pedestal grills

**ASSIGNMENT:** First come, first served

**REGISTRATION:** Self-registration on-site

**FACILITIES:** Vault toilets, boat ramp

**PARKING:** At each site

**FEE:** Tent sites $10; RV sites (with electric and water hookups) $15; double site $16

**ELEVATION:** 7,669 feet

**RESTRICTIONS**

■ **Pets:** On 6-foot leash; take precautionary measures against predators.

■ **Fires:** In fire rings only; charcoal grills permitted; check with campground host, Forest Service office, and postings on the camp bulletin board for restrictions.

■ **Alcohol:** At campsites only

■ **Other:** Quiet hours 10 p.m.–8 a.m.; 15-day stay limit

the campground, but you can take a shower for a $3 fee at Snuffy's Steakhouse and Cowboy Saloon located a mile or so west of the campground on NM 103.

A camp host is always assigned to the RV loop. There is no downed wood here, but the host sells firewood. The Forest Service, New Mexico game wardens, and the Catron County Sheriff's Department patrol frequently, so this campground is extremely safe. Watch children near the roadways and, obviously, at water's edge.

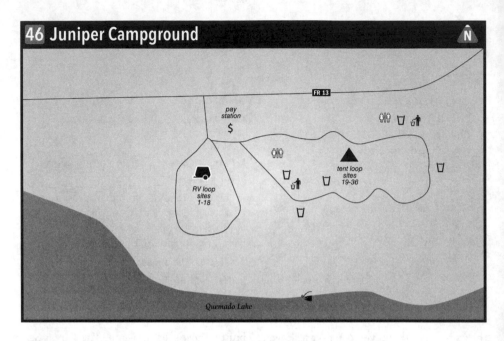

## :: Getting There

From Quemado, follow NM 32 south 14 miles. Turn east onto FR 13 and go 4 miles to the camp.

**GPS COORDINATES**   N34° 8.277'   W108° 29.327'

# 47

# El Caso and El Caso Throwdown Campgrounds

*Tucked back and away from the lake activity, El Caso is a quiet, shady campground.*

**E**l Caso Campground is shaded by ponderosa pine, piñon, cedar, cottonwood and juniper trees. This lovely campground is primitive, with some grassy areas for tents, and slightly to mostly shady, depending on where you set up your tent. Due to its location away from the lake, El Caso experiences less traffic and is more peaceful than nearby campgrounds.

El Caso Campground is divided into four separate areas: El Caso I, II, III, and El Caso Throwdown, which is primarily for equestrian campers. The ground consists of a mix of grass and dirt, and the entry road is dirt. By setting your tent away from the road, your sleeping quarters will escape the dust clouds of passing vehicles. There are no designated numbered sites, so the camping is considered dispersed. RVs can and do utilize this campground, so expect to hear some generator noise. One vault toilet is located just past the campground entrance. Trash bins and potable water spigots are located at Juniper and Pinon Campgrounds. Showers are not provided at the campground but are available for a $3 fee at nearby Snuffy's Steakhouse and Cowboy Saloon on NM 103. Snuffy's is also great if you need a night off from camp cooking.

Forest Service employees work constantly at El Caso, and the Catron County Sheriff's Department and Forest Service law enforcement officers keep a close eye on the campground, so it is secure. You should bring your own firewood or gather wood along the forest roads.

If you feel like stretching your legs, check out the moderately difficult Largo Trail, which is located on the west side of the campground. The Largo Trail traverses grassy fields and passes under ponderosa pines as it climbs toward the El Caso Lookout Tower; it crosses a bridge on the east side of Quemado Lake, so keep an eye out for waterfowl, such as blue herons and osprey. The Largo Trail connects to the Vista Trail, Sawmill Canyon Trail, and Leslie Spring Trail if you want to extend your outing.

## :: Ratings

BEAUTY: ★ ★ ★ ★ ★
PRIVACY: ★ ★ ★ ★
SPACIOUSNESS: ★ ★ ★ ★
QUIET: ★ ★ ★ ★
SECURITY: ★ ★ ★ ★ ★
CLEANLINESS: ★ ★ ★ ★ ★

## :: Key Information

**ADDRESS:** Gila National Forest, Quemado Ranger District, P.O. Box 158, Quemado, NM 87829

**OPERATED BY:** U.S. Department of Agriculture

**CONTACT:** 575-773-4678; www.fs.usda.gov/gila

**OPEN:** Year-round, weather permitting

**SITES:** 22

**SITE AMENITIES:** Parking space, picnic table, fire ring

**ASSIGNMENT:** First come, first served

**REGISTRATION:** Not required

**FACILITIES:** Vault toilets; bring water.

**PARKING:** At each site

**FEE:** None

**ELEVATION:** 7,699 feet

**RESTRICTIONS**

■ **Pets:** On 6-foot leash; this is black bear country and also home to mountain lions, bobcats, and coyotes, so monitor pets closely.

■ **Fires:** In fire rings and pedestal grills only; charcoal grills permitted

■ **Alcohol:** At campsites only

■ **Other:** Quiet hours 10 p.m.–8 a.m.; 15-day stay limit

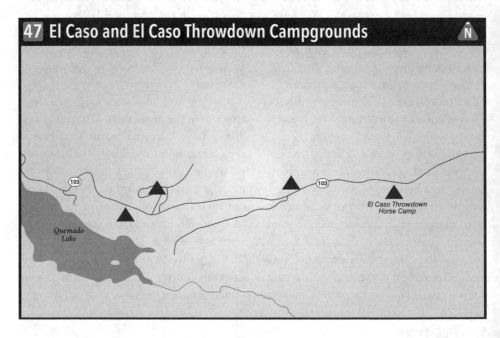

## :: Getting There

West of Quemado, take NM 32 south 14.2 miles to the Quemado Lake/NM 103 sign. At the sign, turn left onto NM 103 and go 4 miles to where Forest Service Road 13 (gravel) begins. Continue straight on FR 13 for 1.4 miles to the campground sign and turn right into the campground.

**GPS COORDINATES**   N34° 8.284'   W108° 27.761'

# 48

# Dipping Vat Campground at Snow Lake

*Frigid Snow Lake is surrounded by mountains and lush green meadows.*

**W**hile **driving** in the Gila Wilderness, my wife, Susan, made the comment, "God has kissed New Mexico, and New Mexico is smiling!" The monsoon seasons are often inconsistent. When they do arrive, they bring this lovely mountain wilderness back to health after a long period of little moisture. Panoramas of lush green ponderosa pine, fir, spruce, and oak forests and meadows filled with wildflowers of myriad colors greet you.

The last 8 miles along Forest Service Road 142 before reaching Snow Lake take you through the horrible destruction of the Bear Fire, which started on June 19, 2006. A campfire out of control was blamed for the devastation. The Bear Fire consumed more than 55,000 acres and raged for more than three weeks. Dipping Vat Campground was spared, as the fire stopped at the western boundary of the camp.

Snow Lake is only 100 water acres at full capacity, but it is beautiful. The lake is surrounded by mountains and lush green meadows. Rainbow trout are stocked here in early spring, summer, and late fall. Snow Lake receives excellent fishing reviews and allows boats with electric trolling motors; it's also excellent for canoeing, kayaking, and inflatable watercraft. The water is cold, and swimming is prohibited.

The lake has two wheelchair-accessible vault toilets, trash bins, a concrete boat ramp, a wheelchair-accessible fishing pier, and a large gravel parking lot. Horse trailers are permitted use of the parking lot by the lake, but pack animals are not allowed in the campground.

Have your fishing license with you at all times because New Mexico Game and Fish wardens patrol frequently and assist the Forest Service with campground security. No campground host is usually assigned here.

Dipping Vat Campground sits a short walk uphill from the lake. Two large loops contain 40 campsites. All sites offer deep grass and are excellent for tents. RV camping is restricted to vehicles under 19 feet in length, and bumpy forest roads discourage most RVs. Sites 1–21 are on a knoll overlooking the lake and have sparse shade. Sites 22–40 sit back farther, fully shaded under a canopy of mature ponderosa pines. Sites are surprisingly large, which is a plus for privacy.

## :: Ratings

BEAUTY: ★ ★ ★ ★ ★
PRIVACY: ★ ★ ★ ★
SPACIOUSNESS: ★ ★ ★ ★ ★
QUIET: ★ ★ ★ ★ ★
SECURITY: ★ ★ ★ ★
CLEANLINESS: ★ ★ ★ ★ ★

## :: Key Information

**ADDRESS:** Gila National Forest, Reserve Ranger District, P.O. Box 170, Reserve, NM, 87830

**OPERATED BY:** U.S. Department of Agriculture

**CONTACT:** 575-533-6232; **www.fs.usda.gov/gila**

**OPEN:** April–Nov., weather permitting; call for road conditions.

**SITES:** 40

**SITE AMENITIES:** Parking space, picnic table, fire ring; some with pedestal grill

**ASSIGNMENT:** First come, first served

**REGISTRATION:** Self-registration on-site

**FACILITIES:** Vault toilets, boat ramp, pier

**PARKING:** At each site

**FEE:** $5

**ELEVATION:** 7,426 feet

**RESTRICTIONS**

■ **Pets:** On 6-foot leash; take precautionary measures against predators.

■ **Fires:** In fire rings only; charcoal grills permitted; check with campground host, Forest Service office, and postings on the camp bulletin board for restrictions.

■ **Alcohol:** At campsites only

■ **Other:** Quiet hours 10 p.m.–8 a.m.; 15-day stay limit

Four pressurized spigots provide water that should be filtered. Three modern, wheelchair-accessible vault toilets are evenly spaced throughout the campground and kept spotlessly clean. Eight varmint-proof trash bins are available throughout camp, and there's plenty of firewood available here.

Warning signs are posted for bears, as well as other wildlife. Mexican gray wolves have been spotted in the Snow Lake vicinity, but there are no known wolf packs of any size near Snow Lake. Howling wolves can occasionally be heard at Dipping Vat, but I was not that fortunate on my visit.

On March 29, 1998, captive-reared Mexican gray wolves were released to the wild for the first time in the Blue Range Wolf Recovery Area, which includes the Gila Wilderness. The goal was a population of 100 animals. Cattlemen protested when the wolves allegedly killed livestock. Twelve wolves were hunted and destroyed by the U.S. Fish and Wildlife Service in 2006. It is estimated that fewer than 25 Mexican gray wolves remain in the Gila National Forest.

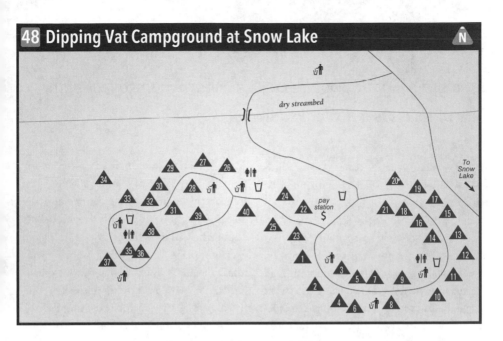

## :: Getting There

From Reserve, take NM 435 south until the pavement ends. This gravel road becomes FR 141. Follow FR 141 past South Fork Negrito Campground to FR 28. Turn south on FR 28 and travel 9.6 miles to a Y and FR 142. Bear left at the Y onto FR 142 and travel 6.6 miles to the campground sign. Turn right at the sign and go 0.2 mile to reach the campground.

**GPS COORDINATES**   N33° 25.383'   W108° 30.057'

# 49

# City of Rocks State Park

*Set among gigantic boulders, some more than 50 feet high,*
*City of Rocks is a geological wonder.*

**M**any southern New Mexico state parks are designed more for RV enthusiasts than tent campers, but the 2,000-acre City of Rocks State Park is an exception. This park, set among gigantic boulders (some more than 50 feet high), is a geological wonder. The rock outcroppings are set in a field of tall prairie grass, with occasional mesquite, scrub oak, yucca, and various cacti. To describe this place in words cannot do it justice, nor can photographs—you just have to experience it for yourself. This is tent camping at its finest in the high-desert environment of the Mimbres Valley.

Pottery shards, arrowheads, and stone tools found here indicate Mimbres Apache tribes inhabited this area between AD 950 and 1200. Several recovered artifacts offer evidence of Spanish conquistadors passing through between 1600 and 1700. Cowboys punched cattle through this area in the 1800s, and in 1953, the movie *The Tall Texan* was filmed here. The state of New Mexico acquired the land and dedicated City of Rocks State Park in 1956.

## :: Ratings

BEAUTY: ★ ★ ★ ★
PRIVACY: ★ ★ ★ ★ ★
SPACIOUSNESS: ★ ★ ★ ★
QUIET: ★ ★ ★ ★ ★
SECURITY: ★ ★ ★ ★ ★
CLEANLINESS: ★ ★ ★ ★ ★

Campsites are named after stars, planets, constellations, and galaxies. The interpretive signs at the entrance and the displays in the visitor center teach guests about the solar system. The park is an excellent place for stargazing, so bring your telescope and star chart. The stars are brilliant here, with no city lights obstructing the night sky. City of Rocks has an observatory at the Orion group site.

The observatory is equipped with a 14-inch Meade LX-200 telescope. They have a star show once a month except during June and July. The entire facility is solar powered, and plans are underway to include a monitor that projects images transmitted through the telescope.

Most campsites are private and set among the boulders, which quells the sounds and activities of other campers. Boulders and juniper and desert willow trees provide surprisingly good shade. Most sites are level, and water runoff is excellent during the rainy season. Tent campers can pitch tents on the gravel areas provided or between boulders. Nearly all sites have trash bins.

The RV area has 10 sites with electricity and water spigots. RVs are allowed to use nonelectric sites, but parking is too difficult at most sites. Generators are allowed but must be turned off by 10 p.m. and cannot be turned on until 7 a.m. Roads are gravel and can become quite dusty when windy. Signs

# :: Key Information

**ADDRESS:** NM 61, Milepost 3, Faywood, NM 88034

**OPERATED BY:** New Mexico State Parks Department

**CONTACT:** 505-536-2800; **www.emnrd.state.nm.us/SPD /cityofrocksstatepark.html**

**OPEN:** Year-round

**SITES:** 45

**SITE AMENITIES:** Parking space, picnic table, fire ring

**ASSIGNMENT:** First come, first served or reserve at **reserveamerica.com** or 877-664-7787.

**REGISTRATION:** At visitor center or self-registration on-site

**FACILITIES:** Restrooms, showers, vault toilets, visitor center, observatory

**PARKING:** At each site

**FEE:** $10; $14 water/electric sites

**ELEVATION:** 5,218 feet

**RESTRICTIONS**

■ **Pets:** On 10-foot leash; take precautionary measures against snakes, bobcats, and coyotes.

■ **Fires:** In fire rings only; charcoal grills permitted; check with campground host, park office, and postings on the camp bulletin board for restrictions.

■ **Alcohol:** At campsites only

■ **Other:** Quiet hours 10 p.m.–8 a.m. (strictly enforced); 21-day stay limit

mandate a 10-mph speed limit within the park. No off-road trails for ATVs or motorcycles exist here—all motorized traffic must remain on the roads.

Four modern vault toilets are strategically located throughout the park. They require a 10-minute walk from the farthest campsites. The well, powered by two windmills, delivers fresh, cool groundwater, which has been treated. The visitor center has a modern comfort station with flush toilets, sinks, and warm-water showers. There is no firewood in the campground; you must bring your own.

A small botanical garden lies near the well at the visitor center, and a larger garden on the south loop road features cacti. Cacti begin blooming in March and continue their colorful show until mid-May. These cactus gardens are a photographer's delight.

The park features several trails open to hikers and mountain bikers. Rock climbing is popular here, but climb at your own

risk. Supervise adventurous children, and remember that the nearest hospital is 26 miles away in Deming. Pay phones are not available at the visitor center, but you might be able to get cellular service here, depending on your carrier.

The best camping seasons are spring and fall. Summertime can produce sweltering temperatures of more than 100°F, but evenings cool into the 70s. Winter temperatures average in the mid-50s during the day but often drop to freezing at night. November sees an increase in park visitors with the arrival of the snowbirds.

Pronghorn antelope, mule deer, wild burros, cottontail rabbits, badgers, bobcats, chipmunks, squirrels, and packrats reside here, and coyotes sing their eerie song nearly every night. More than 75 species of birds reside in the park. Box turtles and various species of lizards also call the park home. Western diamondback rattlesnakes and prairie rattlesnakes are active in the

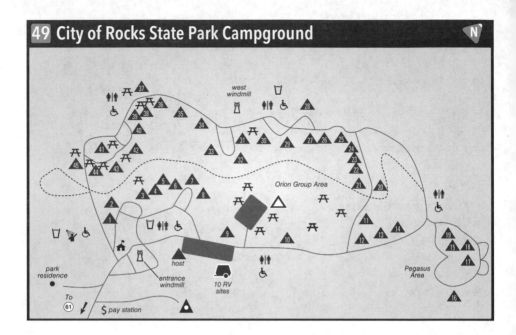

## 49 City of Rocks State Park Campground

warmer seasons, especially at night. When hiking, walk cautiously and avoid wearing shorts; ankle-high hiking boots are recommended. Keep pets leashed and a close eye on your children.

Well-trained and friendly rangers supervise the park and are strict with the rules to ensure a family atmosphere. Rangers are state law enforcement officers, so the security here is excellent.

Nearby, the tiny town of Faywood has a private campground with hot springs. The closest supplies and groceries are in Deming. Rockhound State Park lies 14 miles southeast of Deming and has excellent facilities and a 100-mile view. Rockhound's campground is not tent-friendly due to lack of shade and extremely rocky ground, but it's well worth a visit. Visitors are encouraged to take their treasures home.

## :: Getting There

From Deming, take US 180 north 23 miles. Turn east on NM 61 and travel 3 miles to the park entrance.

**GPS COORDINATES**   N32° 35.282'   W107° 58.462'

# 50

# Gila Cliff Dwellings National Monument:

## UPPER SCORPION CAMPGROUND

*Gila Cliff Dwellings National Monument is a do-not-miss attraction in New Mexico.*

**I**f **there** is one do-not-miss attraction in New Mexico, it has to be the 533-acre Gila Cliff Dwellings National Monument. This national monument was established on November 16, 1907, by President Theodore Roosevelt. The ancient Mogollon (pronounced muggy-own) cliff dwellings are contained inside natural caves on a rugged sandstone cliff. The cave entrances command an incredibly beautiful view facing a vertical mesa covered with coniferous trees. Approximately 180 feet below, the trail meanders along the canyon floor, crosses over a peaceful stream gently trickling by, and then rises through a series of switchbacks to the six caves that comprise the popular archaeological site.

Caves numbered 3, 4, and 5 are fully accessible. Caves 4 and 5 are interconnected. Cave 1 is open, with only the foundation stones of the structure intact. Cave 2 is sealed and not accessible. Cave 6 is closed

## :: Ratings

BEAUTY: ★ ★ ★
PRIVACY: ★ ★ ★ ★
SPACIOUSNESS: ★ ★ ★
QUIET: ★ ★ ★ ★
SECURITY: ★ ★ ★ ★ ★
CLEANLINESS: ★ ★ ★ ★ ★

to access because there were no structures built in this cave and the ceiling is deemed unstable.

Hopi and Zuni tribes claim Acoma ancestry, tracing the migration north and west from this location. Mogollon people lived in these dwellings from 1280 to no later than 1320. The site was occupied by 10–15 families. It remains a mystery why the families abandoned the cliff dwellings after only one generation of use.

Chiricahua Apache are thought to have migrated into this area, although oral traditions of the tribe claim this has always been their homeland. Great warrior Geronimo was born in the 1820s at the headwater of the Gila River, presumably near where the east, west, and middle forks of the Gila River converge (near the visitor center). Chiricahua leaders Mangas Coloradas, Cochise, and Victorio claimed this area as home. The Chiricahua were forced from their homes and into exile in Oklahoma and Florida by 1886.

The visitor center is an essential stop, with a 15-minute video of the cliff dwellings, an impressive bookshop, and souvenirs. The small museum contains artifacts from the Mogollon culture, including pottery and baskets woven from the yucca plant.

The 1-mile trail to the cliff dwellings is a pleasant stroll for the first 0.33 mile, and

## :: Key Information

**ADDRESS:** Gila National Forest, 3005 E. Camino del Bosque, Silver City, NM 88061-7863

**OPERATED BY:** U.S. Department of Agriculture

**CONTACT:** 575-388-8201; www.fs.usda.gov/gila

**OPEN:** Year-round

**SITES:** 10

**SITE AMENITIES:** Picnic table, pedestal grill, fire ring

**ASSIGNMENT:** First come, first served

**REGISTRATION:** Not required

**FACILITIES:** Vault toilet; bring water.

**PARKING:** In lot

**FEE:** None

**ELEVATION:** 5,716 feet

**RESTRICTIONS**

■ **Pets:** On 6-foot leash; dogs not allowed on the Cliff Dwellings Trail; take precautionary measures against predators.

■ **Fires:** In fire rings; charcoal grills permitted

■ **Alcohol:** At campsites only

■ **Other:** Quiet hours 10 p.m.–8 a.m.; 15-day stay limit

then becomes more challenging as it gains elevation. The trail begins its incline over switchbacks to the cliff dwelling site. Allow 1–2 hours for the round-trip. Be sure to carry water, but no tobacco products, trail snacks, or food are allowed on the trail. This is a pack-it-in, pack-it-out trail; there are refuse containers at the trailhead but none on the trail. The trail fee is $3 per person or $10 per family. Pets are not allowed on the trail, but free kennels located behind the trailhead office building are shaded and water bowls are provided. National Park Service rangers and volunteer docents host free guided tours year-round.

The Upper Scorpion Campground is conveniently located just outside the parking lot of the cliff dwellings trailhead. The camp is set against a cliff and adjacent to the road. All 10 sites are walk-in and situated close to the parking lot. The campground has one modern vault toilet. There are no trash bins; you must pack out your trash. Water is available at the visitor center. All sites are shaded, but there is little grass. Some sites are rocky, so bring a good ground pad. There is one parking lot for all campers. The camp is not configured for RVs.

The park opens at 8 a.m. and is locked at 6 p.m. Memorial Day through Labor Day; the rest of the year, hours are 9 a.m.–4 p.m. Only campers and National Park Service vehicles pass this way to the monument, so you will experience peaceful evenings by your fire. The campground is safe, with Park Service officers patrolling the area frequently.

Down the road several miles, Doc Campbell's General Store has adequate grocery supplies, with a few camping items and souvenirs, and showers for a fee.

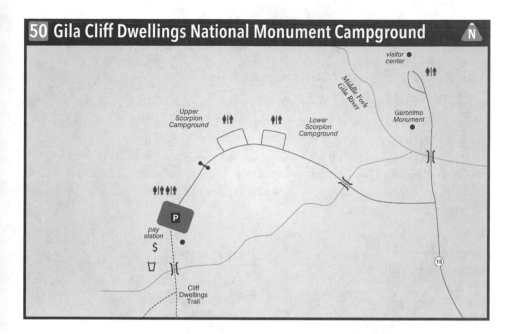

Due to the remoteness of this area, black bears, mountain lions, bobcats, coyotes, and other predators are common, so practice clean camping habits. Be on the lookout for javelinas—a large population of the wild hairy boars live in the Gila Wilderness. Between Lake Roberts and the cliff dwellings, I spotted more than 30 mule deer, with many young fawns among them. Keep your camera ready.

NM 15 traverses some of the wildest and most beautiful country you will ever see, and numerous roadside parking areas provide breathtaking views of the Gila Wilderness.

## :: Getting There

From Silver City, take NM 15 north for 44 miles. There will be a sign directing you to the visitor center. The campground is located to the west of the visitor center.

**GPS COORDINATES**   N33° 13.805'   W108° 15.467'

# APPENDIX A

● ● ● ● ● ● ● ● ● ● ● ● ● ● ● ● ● ● ● ●

## Camping Equipment Checklist

Except for the large and bulky items on this list, I keep a plastic storage container full of the essentials for car camping so they're ready to go when I am. I make a last-minute check of the inventory, resupply anything that's low or missing, and away I go. The simpler you camp, the better. The following list is quite exhaustive but provides a good idea of what might be useful. Clothing, toiletries, and cooler contents will vary by individual and are not included in this list. Many campgrounds profiled in this book do not have water on-site. Always carry an extra 5-gallon water jug.

### COMFORT

Collapsible camping chairs
Fire log
Fire starter sticks
Firewood
Lantern and extra fuel
Toilet paper

### COOKING

Barbecue grill lighter
Campstove and extra fuel
Coffeepot and mugs (Lexan French presses work great)
Dish soap
Dutch oven
Paper towels
Plastic reusable plates
Saucepan
Sauces (Tabasco, liquid smoke, Worcestershire, steak sauce, barbecue sauce)
Scouring pads
Spices (salt, pepper, onion powder, garlic powder, beef and chicken bouillon, sugar or sugar-substitute packets, Parmesan cheese packets, coffee creamer packets)
Skillet
Stockpot
Utensils (knives, forks, spoons, spatula, can/bottle opener, corkscrew)

### FIRST-AID KIT

Ace bandages
Antiseptics
Aspirin or ibuprofen
Band-Aids
Benadryl
Butterfly closures
Compress bandages
First-aid cream
Hydrogen peroxide
Moleskin
Rubbing alcohol
Scissors
Single-edge razor blade
Tweezers

### GEAR BAG

Bungee cords
Carabiners
Duct tape
Flashlights
Rechargeable batteries with car charger
Rope
Tarp(s)

### SLEEPING GEAR

Extra blanket
Ground pad
Pillow
Rubber patch kit
Sleeping bag
Tent
Tent repair tape

## SAFETY

Bear repellent
Compass
Insect repellent
Maps
Small tin with coins for pay telephone
Sunscreen
Whistle

## TOOL KIT

Collapsible shovel
Electrical tape
Extra batteries
Extra tent stakes
Full-size ax
Hand hatchet
Lawn rake
Screwdrivers, pliers, adjustable wrench, wire cutters, needle-nose pliers
Small container of nails
Small roll of baling wire

## WEATHER GEAR

Ball cap
Foil emergency blanket
Gloves
Rain poncho or jacket
Spare pair of shoes
Wool hat

## OPTIONAL FUN STUFF

Bicycles
Bird feeders
Board games
Cards
Digital camera
Fishing gear, bait, and fishing license
Football, Frisbees, sports items
Inflatable raft and paddles, float tube with powered air pump
Mp3 player/portable CD player
Wildlife, birding, and flora identification guides

# APPENDIX B

● ● ● ● ● ● ● ● ● ● ● ● ● ● ● ● ● ● ● ● ● ● ●

## Sources of Information

**COCHITI LAKE DAM PROJECTS OFFICE**
U.S. Army Corps of Engineers
82 Dam Crest Rd.
Peña Blanca, NM 87041-5015
505-465-0307
**www.spa.usace.army.mil/Missions/CivilWorks/Recreation/CochitiLake.aspx**

**SOCORRO FIELD OFFICE (Datil Well)**
Bureau of Land Management
901 S. Hwy. 85
Socorro, NM 87801-4168
575-835-0412
**blm.gov**

**LAS CRUCES DISTRICT OFFICE
(Aguirre Spring)**
Bureau of Land Management
1800 Marquess St.
Las Cruces, NM 88005-3370
575-525-4300
**blm.gov**

**MESCALERO APACHE RESERVATION
(Silver Lake)**
868 Hwy. 244
Mescalero, NM 88340
575-464-2244

**CARSON NATIONAL FOREST**
208 Cruz Alta Rd.
Taos, NM 87571
575-684-2489
**www.fs.usda.gov/carson**

**GILA NATIONAL FOREST**
3005 E. Camino del Bosque
Silver City, NM 88061
575-388-8201
**www.fs.usda.gov/gila**

**LINCOLN NATIONAL FOREST**
3463 Las Palomas
Alamogordo, NM 88310
575-434-7200
**www.fs.usda.gov/lincoln**

**SANTA FE NATIONAL FOREST**
11 Forest Ln.
Santa Fe, NM 87508
505-438-5300
**www.fs.usda.gov/santafe**

**NEW MEXICO STATE PARKS**
1220 S. St. Francis Dr.
Santa Fe, NM 87505
505-476-3224
**www.emnrd.state.nm.us/SPD**

# INDEX

● ● ● ● ● ● ● ● ● ● ● ● ● ● ● ● ● ● ● ● ● ● ● ●

**DEAR CUSTOMERS AND FRIENDS,**

**SUPPORTING YOUR INTEREST IN OUTDOOR ADVENTURE,** travel, and an active lifestyle is central to our operations, from the authors we choose to the locations we detail to the way we design our books. Menasha Ridge Press was incorporated in 1982 by a group of veteran outdoorsmen and professional outfitters. For many years now, we've specialized in creating books that benefit the outdoors enthusiast.

Almost immediately, Menasha Ridge Press earned a reputation for revolutionizing outdoors- and travel-guidebook publishing. For such activities as canoeing, kayaking, hiking, backpacking, and mountain biking, we established new standards of quality that transformed the whole genre, resulting in outdoor-recreation guides of great sophistication and solid content. Menasha Ridge continues to be outdoor publishing's greatest innovator.

The folks at Menasha Ridge Press are as at home on a white-water river or mountain trail as they are editing a manuscript. The books we build for you are the best they can be, because we're responding to your needs. Plus, we use and depend on them ourselves.

We look forward to seeing you on the river or the trail. If you'd like to contact us directly, join in at www.trekalong.com or visit us at www.menasharidge.com. We thank you for your interest in our books and the natural world around us all.

**SAFE TRAVELS,**

*Bob Sehlinger*

**BOB SEHLINGER**
**PUBLISHER**

# ABOUT THE AUTHOR

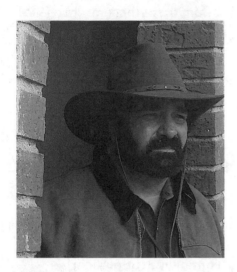

**M**onte R. Parr's outdoor interests were inspired as a child by his grandparents and treks into the San Bernardino Mountains of Southern California. His high school years were spent hiking and camping the hardwood forests behind his family home in Iowa. Monte has lived in California, Iowa, Nebraska, Mississippi, Colorado, and New Mexico. He is experienced in backpacking, backcountry motorcycle camping, and cross-country ski and snowshoe camping. He has camped extensively throughout Iowa, Nebraska, Colorado, Wyoming, and New Mexico.

Monte is an accomplished photographer and is also interested in astronomy, hiking, and fishing. Monte's fascination with Old West history has taken him to dozens of ghost towns, old military outposts, and many ancient American Indian cliff dwellings and ruins throughout New Mexico and Arizona. Monte is a U.S. Air Force veteran; he worked as a ground crew member on C-130 aircraft and is an avid military aircraft historian.

Monte's writing projects include his first book, *Adventures in Camping*, published by Word Productions, Inc. He is also a lyricist and poet and is the creator of Monte's Old West Chuckwagon Spice, a tantalizing barbecue spice that many people love, along with his many camping recipes.

Since moving to New Mexico in 1988, Monte has logged more than 800 nights under the stars, experiencing mountain, desert, and canyon camping throughout New Mexico. He has been a frequent guest on the "ABQ-Connect" radio program for years. Monte is an accounts consultant for a major communications company in Albuquerque, New Mexico. His wife, Susan Parr (also an accomplished author), and dogs Oreo, Goldie, and Koko join him frequently on his journeys. For more on Monte, visit his website at **monteparr.com.**